Yoga's
YAMAS and NIYAMAS

10 Principles for Peace & Purpose

COURTNEY SEIBERLING

ISBN: 1722910208
ISBN-13: 978-1722910204

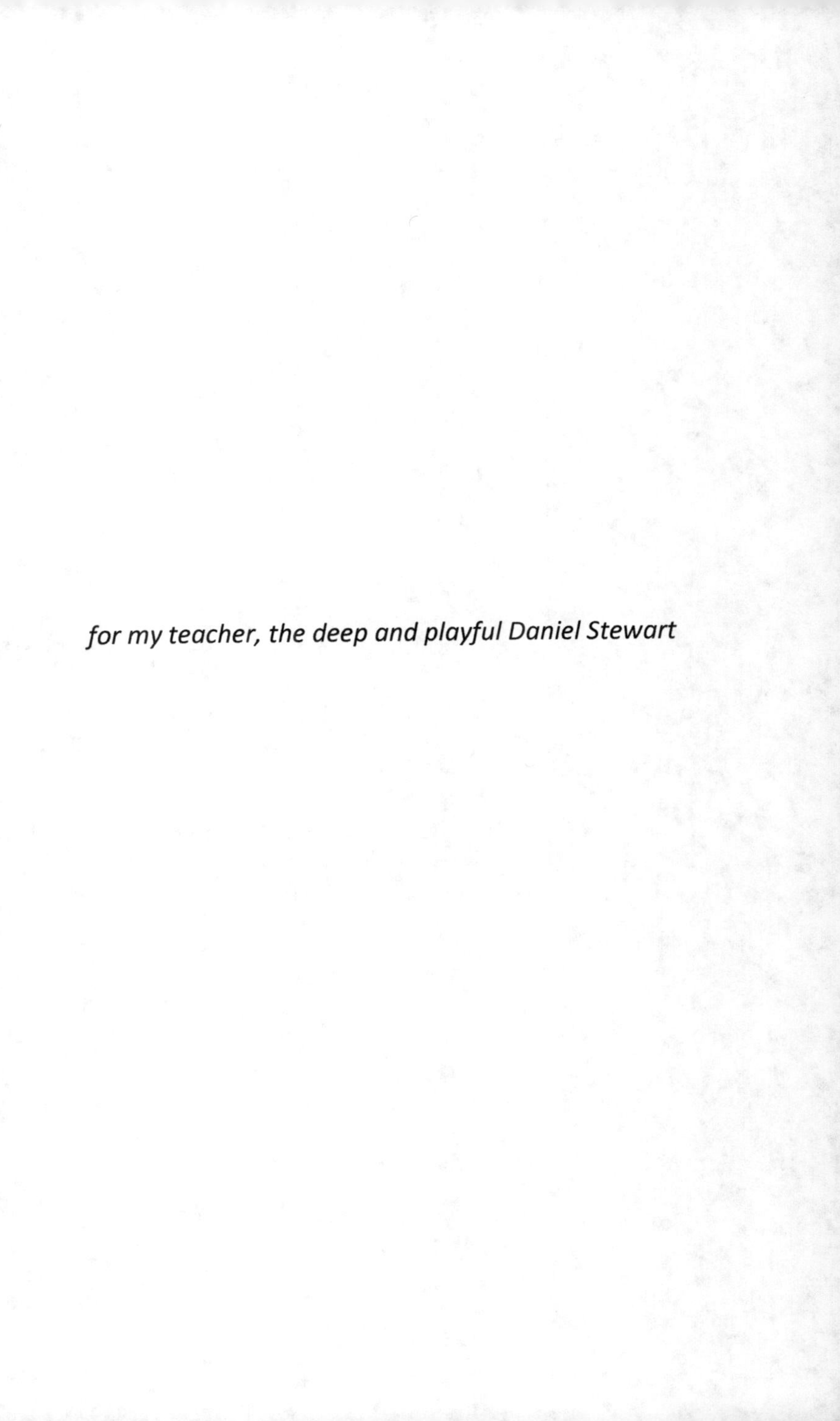

for my teacher, the deep and playful Daniel Stewart

CONTENTS

Why Yoga Philosophy?

Life is beautiful, but it's also hard. Suffering is real. People can be jerks. Injustice abounds. I'm fortunate to live in a country where I'm free to say what I think and do as I please, but the heaviness of things knocks me over sometimes. It can be overwhelming to embrace the world's problems in a big way, so I usually start small, with myself and my actions.

I didn't used to have that maturity. Emotions got the best of me. I treated heartbreak and challenge like enemies, avoided the truth, stayed busy, and tried to make people see things my way. Praying, self-help, running, wine, and Ted Talks helped, but what really stuck for me was yoga.

Like a lot of people, I came to yoga as a form of exercise, but one morning, lying in Savasana, sobbing beneath my eyelids, I realized it was so much more. The cues my teachers gave applied beyond the physical. How I did anything on my mat was how I did everything in my life. If I was being impatient with my body, I was being impatient at work and in my relationships. If I wasn't willing to try new postures, I was in a rut, closed off from opportunities. Yoga became the mirror that showed me what was really going on so I could decide what to do about it.

Patanjali, the author of the Yoga Sutras (the first written yoga text), said yoga is a way to control the mind. I didn't like the word control at first because it sounded harsh and un-yogic, but with time and practice, I've come to understand what he meant. While we don't have control over the way things go, we do have a say in how we choose to respond. Yoga philosophy gives me guidelines to decide the kind of person I want to be in any moment, and my physical practice allows me to experience it in my body. If I aspire to be more patient with other people, I can start on the mat by being more patient with myself. If I've lost my sense of joy, I can find playful approaches to the postures and revive it. I can take any part of the philosophy: letting go, truth, gratitude…and physicalize the wisdom so it becomes like muscle memory. Concepts materialize and become more than ideas. They become active efforts on my mat and then my life.

Yoga means union, the mind and body coming together as one. So often, we use our mind at work and our body for sex and exercise, but the more we can merge the two, the more balanced we feel. When I'm in my body and right mind, aligned with what's true, I can be with my thoughts and other people as they are without excuses or judgement. I am genuine, present, and at peace. Tasks remain important but not immediate. I am able to take on one thing or feeling at a time rather than think I have to figure them all out at once.

The idea is to keep up this union of body and

mind. I detach when I choose to contract and fall into old patterns (*samskaras*), and it happens sometimes. Yoga and life are practices, not things to master. A yoga student of mine once said to me, "You must always be so relaxed and centered all the time because that's how you make me feel." I laughed, shook my head, and told her yoga is the reset button I must press again and again. Stress is an obstacle. Other people are obstacles. Past hurts, projections...wanting to be in control is the king of them. Yoga philosophy has taught me the only thing I have control over is my mind. The days I choose to work on myself and apply the principles that follow are the days I'm at my best. The days I don't, well...thank goodness for that reset button.

What You Should Know

Before I get into the specifics, I want to mention that yoga is not a religion. Lots of religions have borrowed ideologies from yoga, but it's not the other way around. Yoga will only enhance your religious views or offer a spiritual practice if you don't have one.

The *Yamas and Niyamas* are yoga's essential, ethical principles originally mentioned in the Yoga Sutras, the first written explanation of yoga compiled by Patanjali over 2,000 years ago. In the West, yoga is mostly known as a form of exercise, though the Sutras say yoga is an eight-part system working in unison to control the mind. These "limbs" as they are called in the Sutras include the Yamas and Niyamas, breathwork, yoga postures, and various stages of meditation.

The Yamas (how to treat others) and the Niyamas (how to care for yourself) include values such as peace, truth, gratitude, and contentment. When practiced, they make life more manageable and meaningful. Although similar to other moral or religious codes, the Yamas and Niyamas are more freeing than restrictive and a thought process over a hard set of rules. They are basically 10 ways to be a better person.

The Yamas and Niyamas have become the system I use to filter my thoughts and habits through when I'm having a difficult moment or am going through a hard time. When I embody these concepts, I can sit with my feelings, understand myself, and communicate clearly. I'm also more willing to let others be as they are instead of trying to control how I want them to be.

My favorite part of yoga teacher training was our study of yoga philosophy, and the Yamas and Niyamas were what I found to be the most interesting. I couldn't believe these life tip gems had existed for thousands of years, and I'd never heard them mentioned in any yoga class I'd taken. When I went on to teach, I began incorporating the principles in my classes, opening with a reflection on a Yama or Niyama and then sequencing postures that practiced the principle's theme physically. As I searched online for more information about the Yamas and Niyamas, I found descriptions about the concepts but little about relating them to the postures or our daily experiences. I took this as a charge to write the book I wanted. In it, you will find a chapter for each principle explaining what it is as well as a physical yoga practice, consideration, mantra, journal prompt, and a personal account about how I've applied each Yama or Niyama to my own life. In these essays, I step out of the role as a teacher to show myself as a student. It's important you see me as a human, not as someone who gets it right all the time, and how much impact these principles can have.

This book is for anyone who has asked me about my practices, is curious about yoga philosophy, self-improvement, or is seeking more out of life. It is also of value to yoga instructors who want to incorporate philosophy into their teaching or teacher trainees who are deepening their understanding of the first two limbs of yoga. I hope the concepts become relevant and their ancient wisdom wiggles its way into your thinking and choices. There is so much to celebrate and be grateful for, and often all that's needed is a little shift in perspective. These principles offer that shift and are a guide to live life with peace, purpose, awareness, and accountability.

Namaste
(The light in me acknowledges the light in you.)

THE **YAMAS** – HOW TO TREAT OTHERS

The Yamas are five ethical principles from the Yoga Sutras that recommend how to treat others. Through kindness and honesty, we live in peace with our friends and neighbors. By focusing on what we have and give our energy to, life becomes abundant and doesn't overwhelm us. When we let things go, we are free.

Practicing the Yamas makes our interactions and relationships more pleasant, open, joyful, and forgiving. A bonus: we often receive back the qualities we offer.

1 **AHIMSA** – PEACE

Ahimsa is Sanskrit for non-violence and is practiced through peace. (Sanskrit is an ancient Indic language, common of spiritual texts.) Most of us know better than to kill or physically hurt someone, but Ahimsa also considers the way we speak and interact with others. Words and actions can be equally violent. Nasty comments, inconsiderate jokes, or dismissive gestures are destructive to our relationships, reputations, and well-being. Seemingly harmless teasing on the playground may linger and cause shame long after it is spoken. Passive-aggressive behavior can affect an institution's dynamics. What a mother or father tells their child becomes that child's reality. Language is powerful and paralyzes confidence or inspires it.

We are non-Ahimsa-like when our words or actions aren't kind. If we judge a friend rather than try to understand her or become frustrated with a boss's mistake instead of remembering that we've also made them, we are not in the practice of this Yama. Entering situations with demands or acting as though we know best is unhelpful, counterproductive, and no one will like us. Closing off from other viewpoints keeps us from relating, and being short-tempered doesn't do much but increase our stress levels. Reacting aggressively to aggression only makes things more hostile, yet this is often our default setting when we're rattled. It can be difficult to rewire the way we operate, but there is always an opportunity to turn any situation around by making a conscious choice in how we respond. When we speak to others from a calm place, our words are better received and heard. Choosing to be kind can alter a conversation, settle someone down, and create possibilities we never knew were possible.

Ahimsa really begins with the way we treat ourselves, suggesting we offer the same warmth we so freely give to others. We smile and speak kindly to strangers but sometimes don't extend that courtesy to ourselves. We can be harsh when we criticize our appearance in the mirror, forget something, or fail. Some of the things we say to ourselves, we'd never imagine saying to another person! Negative thought patterns clout our reality. What we think, we become. If we doubt our abilities or decide we should be farther in life than we are, we probably won't get much farther, and we certainly won't share the beauty of who we are becoming. The way to love and be loved is to first love ourselves and to be patient with the ebb and flow of relationships.

Caring for our body and giving the mind time to decompress instead of being overscheduled is key. When frazzled or tired, we are often that way with others, but when we make time to nourish ourselves, we tend to be less reactionary. We feel at peace when we approach life from the core of who we are, and establishing a daily grounding practice is a great way to remind ourselves of it. Meditation, yoga, listening to a song, repeating a mantra, breathwork, or anything that centers the mind and reminds us of our body is a way to create peace from within. This gives us stability so the actions of others won't disrupt us.

The concept of Ahimsa also extends beyond our human relationships and makes us mindful of how we treat the environment. Pollution and litter interfere with ecosystems. Excessive water use depletes resources. Overproduction, overdevelopment, even throwing away extra food or using too much toilet paper disregards a world that has already given so much. Animal abuse or the harm of anything affects nature's balance. Ahimsa asks us to be kind to people, plants, animals...ALL things.

To practice Ahimsa, be aware and soften. Ask instead of assume. Listen instead of accuse. Surrender instead of fight. Slow down and respond instead of react. Nurture the body with a breath or a bath and then share the recovered peace with others. Energy is contagious. When we are kind, we are usually matched with kindness. Being mean emboldens others to be mean.

I am amazed time and time again by how much better my relationships are when I approach them tenderly: if I admit I am wrong; when I choose to show up with an open heart instead of my will to be right. Like all the Yamas and Niyamas, Ahimsa is a practice we must recommit to every time we're grumpy, upset, or challenged by a negative thought, comment, or action.

Practice on the Mat

Ahimsa takes a gentle approach to the body. Instead of forcing postures, allow them. Find softness in thought and breath, and share the peaceful nature remembered on the mat, off the mat.

Suggested One-Hour Grounding Asana Practice
A video to practice part of this sequence is available: courtneyseiberling.com/yoga

(All postures are held five breath cycles unless otherwise noted.)

Intention: *Be kind to your body. Take rest as needed.*
Easy Seat: one-minute meditation, slowing down the breath
Ear to shoulder; walk opposite fingers out beyond hip (each side)
Reclined Bound Angle (five breath cycles, pausing at the top and bottom of each breath)
Hug knees to chest, roll knees clockwise and counterclockwise
Rock and roll up to hands and knees
Cat/Cow (repeat five times)
Thread the Needle (each side)
Sunbird to Awkward Airplane (each side)
Plank to Forearm Plank (repeat three times)
Child's Pose
Down Dog
Forward Fold (10 breath cycles)
Mountain Pose
Sun A – arms up, Forward Fold, halfway lift, Forward

Fold, arms up, hands in prayer at heart (repeat three times)
Down Dog
Warrior One (each side)
Warrior Flow – Chair, Forward Fold, halfway lift, Forward Fold, Plank, Down Dog, Warrior One, Warrior Two, Reverse Warrior, Extended Side Angle, Warrior Two, Plank, Down Dog (repeat each side three times)
Yogi Squat – inhale to stand; exhale to squat (repeat ten times)
Wide-legged Forward Bend
Wide-legged Forward Bend Twist (each side)
Legs up the Wall (two minutes)
Hero (two minutes)
Boat (repeat three times)
Cobbler's
Seated Forward Fold
Bridge (repeat three times)
Supported Bridge with Block (one minute)
Reclined Twist (one minute each side)
Reclined Pigeon (two minutes each side)
Star
Corpse (five to eight minutes)

Consideration

Can you be less judgmental or demanding of yourself?

The next time you're angry or annoyed with someone, can you take a breath and choose a kind response?

Mantra

Take a breath. Choose to be kind.

Personal Account

When I found out Donald Trump won the nomination for president, I wanted to punch someone in the face. Preferably him. Any tolerance I'd acquired went right out the window. Throughout running for office, Trump had been flippant, Twitter-furied, consumed by his own popularity, and his campaign seemed like a joke.

NPR streamed on my phone as I lay in bed the night before, listening to the election results come in state by state. I was nervous as it got down to the wire. Pennsylvania and Wisconsin flickered from red to blue to blue to red and at some point, I drifted off to sleep. At three a.m., I woke to a report of "President Elect Trump" and was convinced I was having a bad dream. But as I blinked my eyes open and sat up, I realized the election was over, and it hadn't gone the way my blue, Californian bubble thought it would.

I'm originally from the Midwest, so I know there are different politics and concerns in other regions of the United States, but I couldn't believe some people were this frustrated with the political system, this committed to single-issue voting, or even more terrifying, that some of them wanted Trump to win. I pounded my fists into the pillow, disappointed for Hillary Clinton, who wasn't perfect but a more qualified candidate than Trump. She worked so hard for so long in service to our country, and her resilience to make it this far blew me away. I didn't like that I wanted her to win because she was a woman, but for years, I'd been told a woman could do anything a man could do, and I wanted to believe it. I didn't anymore. Bullying, lying, and "locker room talk" won. Somehow in the year 2016, my fellow Americans voted an unapologetic, misogynistic, egomaniac to the White House, a man who massaged their fears and put on a show of exaggerations with irrational behavior. Or worse yet, many Americans didn't vote at all, too annoyed with politics to bother.

Soon it was mid-November, then mid-December, and Trump's cabinet picks started rolling in: old-fashioned types with politics that felt archaic to me. Backgrounds in white supremacy, deniers of climate change, mostly other businessmen who, like Trump, didn't have any political experience. I kept pinching myself, hoping this was still the same bad dream I'd been having since November, but it wasn't. These appointments were officials who would be in power positions for the next four years (at least).

Other people in my community were outraged, too. My writers' group was spending far less time talking about writing and most of our Thursday nights in therapy/crab sessions together, trying to understand what we couldn't. Arguments and dismay flooded my social media channels. Students at the school where I work asked to play "I hate Trump" songs over the speakers of the cafeteria. (We didn't let them.) The only conversations I had were about how stupid Trump was and how scared he made us all feel. The energy was suffocating. I wanted to fall into a deep sleep for the next four years and wake up when Michelle Obama was president.

Hillary Clinton was handling it better. She appeared to

have moved on, captured in selfies at the grocery store or on hikes with Bill and their dogs. So had Obama. In the final days of his term, I watched my beloved "Yes We Can" president speak gracefully about the transfer of power and his hope for the future because of what he witnessed in service to our country. He encouraged the American people to give Trump a chance. If Obama could with every policy he'd passed in jeopardy of vanishing when Trump stepped in, couldn't I? Yes, I could. Or at least I could try. I had to remind myself that Trump was only one man and decided to alter the way I'd been thinking about him. Maybe he could be the change we needed: a non-politician. An outspoken person. A businessman. Yes, I would give him a chance.

Then came Inauguration Day. I watched Obama shake Trump's hand respectfully before sitting in a row behind the podium. Trump took his place at the microphone and delivered a Mussolini-like address, saying he would restore what had been ruined by the former administration. He talked of taking back power. Of making America what it used to be. Of our nation being the most important one.

I couldn't have been any less inspired by the self-absorbed promises and proclamations, Trump's fist pumping the air as terror pumped through my blood. It was about him, not us. There was no *we* in his wishes. Anger bubbled inside me again, all that intention to reset my thinking gone.

Immediately following the speech, I had to lead a yoga class to a group of distressed, emotionally-charged teenagers. I felt like one of them, and I didn't want to teach. As I entered the classroom, six girls were huddled around a phone replaying Trump's soliloquy and reacting to everything he said with a snarky comment:

Then why do you make all your garments in Vietnam?
How can you hate immigrants if your wife is one?

I wanted to give each of the students a high five and be catty alongside them. I wanted to cancel class. I didn't want to be the calm, love-seeking yoga teacher, and instead, hide out in my office, smash everything, and cry. But when you work at a school, you have to be an adult, no matter how little you feel like one so I took a breath and told the girls to put the phone away and roll out their mats. My original plan for class was irrelevant now, and I inhaled again and searched the room for what we needed. What we needed was to ground ourselves in peace. Not acceptance, but peace. I told the students we were going to open our hearts and breathe. I dabbed rose oil into each of their palms and began. We counted our breaths and released them. We put our bodies into gentle postures that spread our chests wide to the sky and as we did, our hearts filled with love and compassion. I could feel it overtaking the room and was reminded, once again, of the power of the yoga practice. Of the influence steady breath has to reset thinking. Of the control we have over our emotions. I was reminded of Ahimsa.

Ahimsa, peace, doesn't mean we are passive and let things happen to us. It means we center ourselves in what we know to be true and respond in a calm and directed way. Anger is reactive and unproductive. Peace stabilizes intention and creates actual change.

The following morning, I watched as millions of people participated in women's marches across the country and world (750,000 in my city of Los Angeles alone). Individuals came together peacefully to protect civil rights and resist. I watched speeches from my phone and toggled from coverage of the D.C. march to my social media outlets where friends posted their positions from Denver, Nashville, and Los Angeles, responding to what they feared with peace and love. Different ages, races, socioeconomic backgrounds, religions, and genders came together and united. People who had never been in a room together stood together.

I may not have liked the result of the election, but I was inspired by what it made people do: march, call congressmen, volunteer, make donations, start movements... What we don't want to happen can be fuel for what we do, but we must first get out of our reactionary nature and ground ourselves in peace.

***

I was on a hike recently watching yellow-flowered weeds wave and bow in the breeze. In my meditative state, I became aware of a swarm of bees hovering over the part of trail I was approaching. Without much thought, I walked through the cloud of insects, their hum around me like a sandstorm. It was like we were dancing, yet minding our own business, sharing the space of the air. I could see the bees parting one by one to make room for me. I didn't swat. They didn't sting. I breathed and passed through them unharmed. When I cleared the swarm, I stopped and looked back, thinking of Ahimsa, that what we attack forcefully fights us back. What we move through peacefully makes room for faith.

Your Turn (to journal)

What are you fighting against? How can you surrender?

2 **SATYA** – TRUTH

Satya is the second of the Yamas and means truth. There's a lot of buzz in the self-help world about truth, and the word itself can be ambiguous without context, so let's consider it in a specific, personal way. Think about truth as the act of telling the truth. Not only in what you share with others but in what you admit to yourself. I am as guilty as anyone of shying away from feelings I don't like, but uncomfortable feelings (aka the truth) can be signposts to lead us where we need to go next. Reading them can be a battle, but when we acknowledge what's happening in our thoughts and feelings, we embrace who we are and put ourselves on the right path.

It's important to retrain the way we think about feelings. Sadness and anger are often labelled as "bad" and happiness and peace as "good." When we are sad or angry, we're programed to think we need to fix it to feel better, though sometimes sitting in a feeling is the only way to process that emotion, learn something about ourselves, or receive information to make a decision. Acknowledgement is a key element of truth.

The truth is always there, buried underneath our excuses, busyness, or emotional barricades, patiently waiting to be heard. When we ignore what is true, we feel cheated, exhausted, or detached and may not even understand why. We can become bored or depressed if we don't pursue our interests or hide behind the mask of someone we are not. Instead of living in denial or deciding we have no say in our lives, we must look to truth as a friend who encourages us to investigate and act.

Satya is a powerful guide and even when it doesn't know exactly what it wants, it always knows what it doesn't. This is that "trust your gut" feeling we experience when we're in the wrong place or relationship. Sometimes we need to stop and be still to listen to what the truth is trying to tell us. Maybe it's time to move on. We might have outgrown something and shouldn't keep stuffing ourselves into it just because it once fit. Remember being a kid when life would ask great things of you: to start a new school, take the training wheels off your bike, learn how to drive a car, or move away from home? All these challenges kept you engaged and forward-moving. We can lose that push as adults, but life is still ever-changing, and we are ever-evolving. When we try to force things to stay the same, we make no space for what they are now or could be later. Just as a flower grows and blossoms, so should we.

If we get off track, living a life that doesn't feel like who we are anymore, we can get back on course by asking what is true for us now. The answers might be different from what they use to be, but instead of clutching to what is familiar, Satya, truth, encourages us to stay open, receive, and follow our instincts.

When practicing Satya, we pay attention – knowing and owning our feelings no matter how much they put our lives in conflict. We are not in conflict with ourselves though, because we are in harmony with our heart. Being aligned places us in jobs and relationships that feel meaningful and give us a sense of purpose. It's easy to confuse a job or relationship where we're needed with one we need. Being needed can make us feel important but deplete us of the energy we should give our own pursuits and dreams. The better we get at making choices that reflect our interests, the more we'll find opportunities that excite us and the less dramatic our life transitions will be.

I hope I'm not scaring you by making truth sound like a battle. Satya isn't always a struggle. Sometimes the Universe nudges us along naturally. When it's easy and right, all we must do is say, "YES, YES, YES!" and follow.

So how do we do it? How do we live authentically? We practice Satya by committing to who we are. Only you can be you, and only I can be me; no one else can laugh or sing or tell a story in the way we each do – it's attractive to let ourselves be known. Think of someone you love. More than likely, you've seen them goofy and fragile, and they've probably experienced the same of you. We feel connection when we're able to witness others as they really are. If we try to imitate or live up to an ideal of how we think we should be, we aren't letting ourselves be our ideal version. I had a writing teacher who said writers waste their talents trying to sound like other writers – that when we strive to be like the greats, we miss sharing our own greatness.

Another component of Satya is valuing honest communication and discouraging gossip. This means we don't say something until we know it to be true, and we don't withhold information to protect someone. The truth will always surface and hurt more if we aren't upfront about our feelings from the beginning. Telling the truth doesn't mean we flippantly throw our emotions at others, however. We work to understand why we feel the way we do and then share it. We involve our loved ones in our concerns and insecurities to establish a system of trust and support. When we speak from the seed of our truth, even if what we have to say is not what others want to hear, we plant ourselves in their hearts because they feel our desire to be understood. When we mean to be seen, we usually are.

Practice on the Mat

Satya is practiced physically by finding an individualized expression of each yoga posture. Listen to what is true for the body and respond appropriately.

<u>Suggested One-Hour Asana Practice Taking Variations of Each Posture</u>
A video to practice part of this sequence is available: courtneyseiberling.com/yoga

(All postures are held five breath cycles unless otherwise noted.)

Intention: *Let your expression of each posture reflect how you feel in that moment, using modifications or taking an advanced version if it is available.*

Easy Seat: *How you are feeling in your body, mind, and heart?*
Cat/Cow (repeat five times)
Sunbird – elbow to knee (repeat each side three times)
Child's Pose (Stay if more rest is needed or...)
Down Dog
Forward Fold
Mountain Pose
Moon – side to side (repeat three times)
Sun A – arms up, Forward Fold, halfway lift, Forward Fold, arms up, hands in prayer at heart (repeat three times)
Crescent Salutations (with knee down or up) – arms up, Forward Fold, halfway lift, Forward Fold, Plank, Down Dog, Crescent, Plank, Down Dog (repeat each side three times)
Sun B – Chair, Forward Fold, halfway lift, Forward Fold, Plank, Down Dog, Warrior One, Plank, Down Dog (repeat each side three times)
Standing Pigeon (each side)
Tree (each side)
Legs up the Wall
Shoulder Opener on Belly – arms in T, roll to the side (one minute each side)
Sphinx
Superman
Seated Twist (each side)
Cobbler's
Double Pigeon (one minute each side)
Seated Forward Fold
Easy Seat: *This relaxed open state is who you are, not the stressed out parent or the person who snips at her sister. For the next three minutes, sit in your true self.*
Corpse (five to eight minutes)

Consideration

Can you think before you speak and make sure what you share with others is true?

Mantra

Tell the truth.

Personal Account

I broke someone's heart. Badly. Someone who trusted me. Who loved me. Who did everything with me in mind. I spent the final months of our relationship trying to recover a mistake I made of not being honest about what I wanted from the beginning. By the end, I didn't even know what I wanted. I focused so much on accommodating his desires and dreams to make our relationship work that I forgot about my own.

When we met, I was planning to leave Los Angeles, and he'd just moved back. I came to LA to be an actor, which I wasn't anymore, and was annoyed it had become so expensive and overcrowded and had driven all my friends away. His nearest and dearest were natives of the city, and he had recently taken a position at a company that was perfect for him. Because I was excited about the potential of us, I ignored my LA fatigue and decided to stay so we could have a real chance at a relationship. After a few months of dating, I was so sure, so deeply in love that I announced we should move in together, and he and his parents suggested we buy a house instead of rent. They had lots of money. I had none. It felt wrong to buy something since I wanted to leave LA and couldn't contribute, but I kept my mouth shut, and we started perusing open houses on weekends.

Just as my boyfriend had swept me off my feet when we met, the idea of playing house carried me through months and months of looking and a year later, we closed on a property. It was a beautiful home in a trendy neighborhood with tall ceilings and lots of light, but it didn't feel like me. It was modern like his childhood home and not the quaint, single-family craftsman I kept falling in love with in a different neighborhood. But the modern house was a good investment and had a rental unit that would pay for our entire mortgage if we did it right. I'd never been good with money and had a lot to learn. We moved in and hosted a housewarming and our friends and families came to celebrate with us. People told me how lucky I was, but I kept waking up bathed in the speckled light of our bedroom and feeling exposed. It didn't look like my house or my life. I'd completely abandoned my bohemian style of living. In the same week we moved, I also quit my job of eight years to run the rental unit attached to the house. This was also at the suggestion of my boyfriend and his parents and meant I'd be making less money and leaving my professional life, but it would give me more flexibility in the day to write, which is what I wanted to do, so I decided to try it.

I thought loving my boyfriend was reason enough to change how I was living, but it left me hollow and anxious. I missed the bustle of my work community. I swallowed secret desires to move back to New York to be with my best friends. Even though I had an abundance of time to write, I spent it cleaning and grocery shopping to contribute to the household, and it seemed like the only way I could. My boyfriend asked none of this of me and insisted I stop cleaning and start writing, but I couldn't. I felt like a maid and convinced myself that all the neighbors thought I was a Stepford wife who had no real goals for her own life other than to appease and tend to her man.

I was angry and grumpy and didn't know how I'd become either of those things. I'd been bratty during the house-hunting process and hadn't understood why. Anytime a doubt or concern surfaced, I kept it to myself because I didn't want to disrupt the forward movement in my relationship. In small ways, I tried to express I wasn't ready for a house and was uncomfortable with the gift my boyfriend's parents had given him for the down payment, but he reassured me he couldn't pass it up – a house was smart for our financial future, and he was doing this for me. But why didn't my feelings matter? Why was the best decision for us...his? My boyfriend and his dad were calling all the shots. It was their money, but it was frustrating to spend afternoons looking at houses and then listen to my boyfriend talk to his dad about what we were going to do about them. I didn't feel like his partner, but I didn't say it. Saying it was like asking him to choose between his family or me, and I didn't want to put him in that position. He loved his family, and I loved him. I worried the house was a prognostication of how other big decisions in our life would go, and I wanted us both to have the futures we wanted.

I started to get quiet and pushed away from my boyfriend to process why I was feeling so conflicted. He noticed and tried to pull me back. I felt suffocated and alone and then one morning as he was getting ready for work, I revealed everything: the decisions I made had been based on his happiness and not mine; I didn't want the house because I didn't want to live in LA; I needed to know if I wanted to move somewhere else, we could. I told him I struggled to connect to his family, who were a huge part of our lives, and even though I cared about them very much, I couldn't figure out how to make them my own. I didn't think I wanted to have children, and I knew he very much did. I said I was uncomfortable about our financial differences and outlooks, that our dissimilar attitudes and approaches toward life made me nervous. I spewed it all: months and years of opinions buried deep that I didn't even know I had until I started listening to myself. Everything I said put my boyfriend and me in conflict. My greatest fear of separating us was coming true — his future was headed one way and mine was headed the other. I didn't want to bring any of it up because I didn't want anything to get in the way of my love for him, but I'd gotten in the way of loving myself.

Discussions about our differences went on for weeks. He was patient and loving, giving me space when I needed to think and listened when I needed to be heard, but I'd built up so much resentment toward him that it felt irreversible. While he was willing to work with me to fix what had been broken, the reality of what I needed to do was becoming more and more apparent.

Then I made it worse. I told him I was attracted to someone else. A man had taken my yoga class, and I felt a surge of interest and curiosity. My boyfriend didn't like hearing this obviously, suspecting something physical had transpired between me and my student. It hadn't, and most people keep quiet about crushes like this, but in the theme of the truth I'd been telling, I didn't want to hide anything anymore. My boyfriend refused to discuss any of our other issues. He stopped listening, and the only thing on his mind was this other guy. He needed to know he was the only man I'd ever want. I needed to know we were partners, and I could be open with him. We were fighting different fights, and I could see the truth creeping around our house, peering in the windows, neither of us brave enough to let her in.

And then one day I did. I let the whole truth inside. I was alone, mopping the floor, and felt her on the other side of the door. I opened it and allowed truth to sweep through our house and fill me with a terrible relief. She told me what I had to do.

While my boyfriend was on a business trip, I moved my stuff out. I emptied drawers I'd just filled. I wrapped my mugs in fliers addressed to the house we'd looked so hard to find. I took my books off the shelves, and I separated our records.

The afternoon of my boyfriend's return, I paced the living room, searching for what I was going to say, and sobbed on the dining room floor. Our love story was not supposed to end this way. We both had big hearts, and he was the best person I'd ever met. I thought about our courtship: the dance parties in living rooms, adventures to National Parks and county fairs, wine country, and Asian markets. I remembered the way he held me in the morning before I got up, how he could fix anything with his hands, the flowers he picked and assorted for me from other people's yards, and how I was dissembling it all with my decision. When it was time to retrieve him from the airport,

I pulled myself up from the floor, slid keys from the top of my cleared-out desk, and turned to look at the house. It was so empty and sad, and I couldn't believe this is what he was coming home to after he'd loved me and bought it to make me happy.

It was like starring in a bad movie as I descended the stairs to the street and waved to a neighbor like it was a normal day. I got in the car and was too dizzy to drive so I traced the steering wheel to focus my attention. I tried to talk myself out of leaving, but how would I explain the empty house? I decided not to think, but that only made me think harder. And then, I just turned the key in the ignition and began the scene I didn't want to end.

At the airport, I waited on a bench, searching the sky for a sign to appear and tell me I was doing the right thing, but no sign came. Looking up made me feel small, and I thought of that Joni Mitchell song where she says we are all made of stardust which usually reminds me of how insignificant my problems are, but this felt really significant. I was about to leave someone I loved and not have a job or a place to live.

My boyfriend texted he'd landed and after a few minutes of pause, passengers exited the terminal in twos and threes and gathered around the baggage carousel. I didn't know where to look so I kept my head down until I saw my boyfriend's tan coat and buoyant outline. I lifted my chin and showed my face, and he threw his bag from his shoulder and ran to me. He took me in his arms, asking what was wrong, but I didn't want to tell him because I didn't want my whole life to change. I motioned we should walk away from the crowd, and when we reached the parking garage, he asked again. I looked at him with so much guilt I thought it would stop both our hearts.

He took my shoulder in his large hand and demanded I tell him what it was, and I said, "I don't think you're the right partner for me."

His face changed. He released me from his comfort, and I knew I'd never feel it again.

We sat in the car like strangers as he stared out at the tarmac with glassy eyes that had once only held love for me. I knew there was nothing more to say and started the car to drive us home – to his home, to the one I'd cleared my stuff of. He didn't offer to drive like he usually did. He didn't put his hand on my thigh like it always was. There was traffic and evening news helicopters buzzed above, and we crawled down the freeway, the smog putting a layer of heavy muck on what was already so weighted.

The weeks that followed were agonizing, like an actual sword was twisting in my side at any moment. I hated the truth. I didn't want it to be the source of so much pain for us both and spent my time searching for a new job and a place to live and reading his texts in-between: angry...sad...at peace...longing...a wash of wanting me back and never wanting to see me again. I felt all these ways, too. I accepted the words he cut me with no matter how much they hurt. I tried to stay calm and convince myself this is what I wanted. I rented a storage unit and slept on a friend's couch and told myself it wouldn't be like this forever but those long nights felt like they were my forever. Every time I had the inclination to drive over to the house and say, "I'm sorry," and beg for him to take me back so we wouldn't have to be in so much pain now, I reminded myself it would be better later if I didn't.

After a couple of weeks, I asked if I could pick up a few things I'd left behind and suggested we talk. I went over to the house on a Sunday morning, and he made breakfast. He couldn't look at me and kept his hands busy, chopping and mixing and flipping while I plucked blueberries from a carton and popped them into my mouth. I ran my fingers over the beautiful, green Europly countertop that would never be mine again, knowing he would never be either. He made jokes to lighten the mood as things sizzled on the stove, but when we sat down to eat, he couldn't avoid my eyes anymore. He was done for. I was done for. We both cried and held hands over the table. But we were done-in differently. He wanted me to come back to him. I wished I hadn't had to leave.

After breakfast, I collapsed over the sink, overcome with sadness and hatred toward myself for abandoning him and our house and the life I was unmaking. He held me as I heaved inside my sobs, and his fingers fell in my hair gently, the way he always was with me. I stayed between his chest and chin for as long as I needed, as he said my name with the familiarity of someone who knew me better than I knew myself. When I broke from the embrace, he asked if I'd make love to him one last time. I looked in his eyes, comfortable and safe, the ones that had held me through so much, not wanting to reject him again. Linen-scent wafted from the laundry exhaust, overpowering the haze of almond cleaner I'd bought to make a memory of how our house would smell. He'd mopped. He knew I liked things spotless, and he was always thinking of me. Now, he was asking me for something he needed, and I couldn't give it to him. It wasn't the right thing for me. He wasn't the right man for me. This was my truth.

***

This is the longest essay in the book. I didn't pare it down to the length of the others because admitting my feelings about a future with this man was the hardest personal work I've ever done. Hurting someone I loved that much was awful. The guilt still lingers. Loneliness and uncertainty were constant visitors of my new apartment, and I couldn't seem to move on with anyone else. I kept clutching to the truth, trusting it knew more about my future happiness than I did, and I confided in this principle. Even though our love seemed boundless, my boyfriend and I hadn't aligned on what mattered: family, money, lifestyle, and communication. The deeper I buried these realities, the messier they were to dig up, but finally acknowledging, embracing, and owning what was in my heart gave me the courage to honor it. Even with all I lost, I found the deepest love and respect for myself.

Your Turn (to journal)

What are you lying to yourself about?

3 **ASTEYA** – GRATITUDE

If there's one take away from this book or you're seeking a feel-better shortcut without having to apply much effort, practice gratitude. Gratitude, or *Asteya* as it is called in the Yamas, is the single-handed most significant way to transform your life. Being grateful reveals the beauty and fortune already present, and practicing Asteya filters out deficiencies so life appears abundant without changing anything externally. Our experiences and relationships shift when we alter the way we see them, and we stop wishing for what we don't have because we feel glad for all we do.

When we're down or going through something hard, it can be annoying to hear, "Just be grateful!" but choosing to be can pull us out of despair. Getting fired could lead to a better job. Being sick makes us appreciate feeling well. Jealousy often provokes desire and action. The Yoga Sutras say it's possible to control the mind by choosing behaviors wisely. Asteya places the focus on what we have, and being grateful welcomes more good into our lives. Instead of seeing the cup as half-empty; it's overflowing, and we decide to be happy now instead of think, *I'll be happy WHEN...* Even when life is dismal, we find blessings in having our basic needs met: running water, shelter, food, the ability to read, or a friend who will listen.

Think about the people in your life. Are there some you look forward to seeing and others you dread? I have a vendor at work who is whiny and ungracious. He constantly complains about not receiving enough business from the community, and whenever he calls or stops by, my body tenses. Another vendor I use has a can-do attitude, a great sense of humor, and is always so thankful for the work I give him. Gratitude is energizing, and being around grateful people makes us feel generous and joyful.

Asteya is the "Seize the day!" of the Yamas, reminding us to treat each moment as sacred. If you've ever lost a loved one, your perspective changes. Just this morning, I received news that a co-worker of mine suddenly stopped breathing and died at the age of 59. The stress and pettiness I was carrying dissipated, and I couldn't do anything but sit in my car and watch myself breathe. The trees outside my window loosened their hold in the wind, and I was overcome with how beautiful the street was. I'd parked there so often and never noticed. The errands I planned to run no longer mattered, and I wanted to fill my day with something meaningful. I called friends and spent the afternoon laughing and crying with them. I felt so fortunate to be alive, acutely aware it could all be taken away at any moment.

Some translations of this Yama say that Asteya is non-stealing. Most of us know better than to shoplift or hijack a car, though we can steal energetically from others without realizing it. When we interrupt someone in conversation, we imply our thoughts are more important. If we dominate a group project, we miss out on the insights other people may have. Calling a friend and launching into a rant or charging into a co-worker's office without asking if she has a moment to listen disregards others' time. Imagine how much more pleasant our interactions would be if we approached people considerately instead of in a self-serving way. Have you ever felt intruded upon or disrespected? It triggers a reluctance to help. But when asked if available to assist, there's often a willingness to be of service. We should practice giving what feels good to receive.

We can also steal from ourselves by offering more energy than we have to give. When we take on too much work or commit to social obligations we don't have time for, we drain ourselves. We can't expect to work a full-time job, be a present parent, keep the house clean, prepare home-cooked meals, sleep eight hours a night, practice yoga every morning, and volunteer regularly at a non-profit. Something needs to give. Accomplished and depleted aren't a pretty pair. Being busy doesn't equate to living fully. Working hard is admirable, but when this is our identity, we ignore a greater identity, which is the connection to everything around us: the sun on our face, shared laughter, or a lover's touch.

Asteya can be practiced in small ways. We can say thank you more. We can leave work on time instead of staying late so we have the evening to recharge. We can listen to a friend without thinking of our own agenda, or be more conscious about the amount of food we pile on our plate or how many paper towels we use. When we do, we realize how little we need. We can also be less demanding of our relationships. The people in our lives are there to enhance and support us but not be our sole source of happiness or what holds us up every day. We are all responsible for our own well-being, and while it is beautiful to have deep and meaningful relationships, we can only expect so much from them. When we appreciate people for who they are, our relationships aren't suffocated and can be a healthy exchange of experiences.

Asteya is a small shift that makes a big difference. Take a minute to acknowledge you are alive and what a miracle that is. Feel your heartbeat. With your heart, you can love and be loved. With a functioning mind, you can think and learn whatever you want. You can be whoever you choose, and you can always keep choosing. You are not what you do but how you do it. How will you revere this next moment?

Practice on the Mat

To actively practice Asteya, be grateful on the mat. Discover what the body can do, and treat it with deep appreciation. Make the most of the time available to breathe and move.

<u>Suggested One-Hour Heart Opening Asana Practice</u>
A video to practice part of this sequence is available: courtneyseiberling.com/yoga

(All postures are held five breath cycles unless otherwise noted.)

Intention: *Instead of criticizing what your body can't do, be grateful for what it can.*
Cobra (repeat five times)
Sphinx
Cat/Cow (repeat five times)
Sunbird (each side)
Thread the Needle (each side)
Child's Pose
Down Dog
Forward Fold
Sun A – arms up, Forward Fold, halfway lift, Forward Fold, arms up, Cactus arms (backbend), arms up, hands in prayer at heart (repeat three times)
Sun B – Chair, Forward Fold, halfway lift, Forward Fold, Plank, Down Dog, Warrior One, Plank, Down Dog (repeat each side three times)
Chair Twist (each side)
Crescent to Crescent Twist to Lizard (each side)
Down Dog
Dancer (each side)
Legs up the Wall (two minutes)
Hero with Shoulder Opener (one minute each side): *Think of something you are grateful for and let it fill your heart.*
Cow Face (each side)
Camel (repeat two times)
Superman (repeat two times with cheek down to rest between sides)
Bridge (repeat three times)
Reclined Twist (each side)
Happy Baby
Single Pigeon (two minutes each side)
Reclined Bound Angle (three minutes)
Corpse (five to eight minutes)

Consideration

Whenever you experience a tinge of jealousy or feel as though you're lacking something, can you think of something you are grateful for?

Mantra

What DO you have?

Personal Account

I used to be very judgmental of recreational drugs. I prided myself on being an open-minded person, but I HATED when my friends used substances. I avoided parties in college if drugs were the focus and left at the sight of them while dabbling in New York City nightlife as a young adult. I hadn't known anyone who overdosed or messed up their life because of addiction, so it was confusing why I was so overcome with anxiety, but my feelings were intense. I suffered panic attacks, convinced a classmate or boyfriend might die suddenly if she or he tried something even once, and the worry physically manifested in my body.

In my late 20s, I went to Coachella, a music festival near Los Angeles known for its lavish parties. My boyfriend of this decade had rented a house near the grounds with some of his friends, and the music lineup was so good I decided to tag along. The house was on a golf course and had wide rooms, thick pillars, and an ornate pool. It reminded me of the set of one of those celebrity reality shows, and I was completely out of my element. The group allotted one of the three bathrooms for cocaine and the dining room table for pills...mushrooms...things I'd never seen...all strung out like a mess of tangled Christmas lights. Housemates grabbed one of this and one of that and washed down their selections with a beer or a shot of whiskey at 10 a.m., 3 p.m., or long after I put myself to bed. I tried to ignore the activity around me and remember the bands I came to see, but I couldn't, and the weekend exhausted me and my relationship. I lost trust in my boyfriend because he didn't ease my uneasiness. I became an outsider as he slipped from a person I loved to one I didn't recognize. I was aggravated drugs were at the center of the weekend and not the music, and I left Coachella alone early, thinking other people had ruined my experience of the festival.

I started seeing a therapist to try to understand why I let the choices of others get the best of me. I couldn't handle the carefree nature of the people I spent time with at that house, and I wasn't able to sleep if I was home and my boyfriend was out at night without me. I was convinced he was on a cocaine binge even if I knew he was at band rehearsal, and the thought of him going back to Coachella ate me up. I was mature enough to know my discomfort was about me and not him, but I couldn't understand why I allowed it to create such distance between us.

Eventually, my boyfriend left me for someone who loved him for who he was and didn't judge him for what he did. This made me feel stupid, but I was relieved not to have to go to parties anymore or be anxious about what may or may not happen on the weekend. I wouldn't admit it in all my broken-heartedness, but I knew I was better off without him.

And yet...breaking up didn't make my anxiety go away. A year later as Coachella approached, I knew my ex-guy and his new girlfriend would attend, and he'd have fun with her in a way he hadn't with me. I was jealous and upset I couldn't be a more relaxed and fun person, and I turned into a basket case. I paced my studio, scared for my ex-boyfriend and his girlfriend and had terrible daydreams one of them would overdose. The pit of my stomach had a never-ending ache in it, and chunks of my hair were falling out and collecting in the shower drain. As my mind spun out of control, I fed it by spending all my free time on Facebook, stalking for evidence that my worries about the upcoming festival were valid.

I needed to stop looking at social media and leave the house, so I took long walks and tried to keep busy. I saw friends and went to yoga and yelled out to the Universe for relief from the awful feelings I was experiencing.

I was in a department store when I received a response. While trying on clothes, John Denver's *Take Me Home, Country Roads* came on the radio, a song my dad used to play on guitar when I was growing up. He died when I was 16, and it comforts me to hear the music he covered which always seems to find me when I need a nudge of encouragement. In that dressing room moment, surrounded by the chorus, I felt grateful for my healthy body. I looked at the curves, scars, and softness of my arms, hips, and belly in the full-length mirror and realized the distress I had about my ex wasn't about him treating me poorly. It was about me wanting to treat my body with the utmost respect. Because I'd seen my father's once healthy body taken by illness, I couldn't make sense of battling mine for fun. From an early age, I had gratitude for my brain and organs that was rare of people my age. There was nothing wrong with me, nor was there anything wrong with my ex-boyfriend. We just had different experiences which led us to different lifestyle choices. I felt a surge of appreciation for all those uneasy years with my boyfriend. They showed me what I cared about and the way I wanted to live.

Now at 36, I'm still amazed by all my body can do and how hard it works to function. It's starting to age, and with every wrinkle or sag, I remind myself I'm still beautiful, even more so for the years I've been granted on this earth. Failures and obstacles have made me more aware and mature. Laughter and sunshine have marked my face. Any time I remember, I find gratitude for something I've gained instead of something I've lost, and this is what I choose to see reflected in the mirror.

Your Turn (to journal)

For the next ten minutes, make a list of what you are grateful for.

4 **BRAHMACHARYA** – MODERATION

Brahmacharya translates as celibacy. Keep reading, I'm not going to ask you to give up sex! This Yama is the most difficult to relate to in the Western world, though contemporary yoga scholars describe it as a mindful approach to the way we distribute our energy. Before discussing the modernized view, however, it's essential to understand the principle's origin. Some religious and spiritual practices recommend seekers take vows of celibacy to focus on their relationship with a higher self. Sexual energy can be distracting and depleting when misdirected, and it's thought that by preserving and channeling sensations into a focused form like meditation, control can be gained over the mind. Patanjali discusses the benefits of this regulation in the Yoga Sutras, suggesting the mind serves as either a doorway or a barrier to our perception of reality. If we want to free ourselves from being enslaved by thoughts, we shouldn't let impulses boss us around. Pausing, acknowledging instincts, and deciding what to do moderates our actions so we're more aware of our options.

When we control how we expend energy, we don't exhaust ourselves. Restraint helps us find balance so we don't spiral out of control and gives a hierarchy of what to do when. We learn we *have* feelings but are not the feelings themselves. Instead of letting emotions control our behavior, we use them as information to decide what's deserving of our energy and what to let alone.

Brahmacharya tempers stimulations and distractions. We are pulled in many different directions during the day as our devices ding and demand our attention. By curbing our reactionary nature, we can manage time so we're not so immediate about everything. What we give our energy to is what grows. If a supervisor barks an overwhelming amount of assignments at us, we can react with panicked energy and try to complete every task as it's requested, or we can write down what needs to be done and prioritize the work. If someone cuts us off in traffic, we can throw up a finger and yell, or we can take a breath and not allow the act to take too much of us. We can set aside time for projects and refrain from checking email during these reserved blocks in order to get things done.

Time is precious. If we aren't careful, we can get off track and find ourselves in the wrong job, give energy to negative thinking, or surround ourselves with people who aren't good for us. We may talk ourselves into doing things we think we should do instead of what we want to do or become lost in the ideas of a dream instead of working hard to bring dreams to life. Intention is powerful and a practice of Brahmacharya channels it mindfully so we make the most of our time. Following our heart, trusting our gut, and being honest about what we want keeps us engaged in meaningful activities. Awareness of thinking patterns and what we choose to believe is key. Our thoughts become our reality. If we give attention to how things were in the past, our habits and life remain stuck and unchanged. If we are present and aware of how events change us, we evolve.

In our fast-paced lives, even if we are doing something we love, we can be tricked into thinking more is more and that we must complete as many tasks as possible as quickly as we can. This pattern causes us to rush to produce. But of what quality? Of what joy? Have you ever compared an artisan's craftsmanship to that of a mass-produced, machine-made product? You see the time taken in the stitches and quality. You can taste the love in a home-cooked meal. You feel your worth if someone sits with you and doesn't look at their phone. We brag about our ability to multitask, but when we do more than one thing at once, we don't really give our attention to anything. At the high school where I work, students constantly tell me how much they have to do and how overwhelmed they feel. This is a real problem, and the administration has noticed a spike in anxiety and depression. I remind students they can't study for math, practice scales, write college essays, and watch Netflix at the same time or even in the same night. The only way to do it all is to do one thing at a time. Brahmacharya is a mindfulness exercise and a commitment to presence so we fully engage in whatever task we are doing.

Sensitivity to mental and physical states is essential to the practice of this Yama. Some days we wake up full of energy and inspiration. Other days, we are unmotivated, sick, or sad. We must honor and know where we are emotionally and physically and respond with an appropriate level of ourselves. Doing check-ins each morning helps to differentiate our fluctuations of energy. Some days, the best thing to do may be nothing. Other times, it's good to push ourselves to file our taxes, exercise, scrub the stove, or meditate. Life is a mixture of work and play, connection and seclusion.

Even in this contemporary view of Brahmacharya, there is still a benefit in considering its sexual origin. I use Brahmacharya as a tool for sexual responsibility so I'm thoughtful about who to give this intense, intimate energy to and when. Instead of using sex to gain power, comfort, or temporary relief, I value it as a meaningful act. It is an extension of myself, a way to express connection, or a creative union of energies if I want to make a child.

Brahmacharya monitors impulses, feelings, and passions so we move toward what we want with accountability and balance. Not giving too much or too little, we mindfully walk the tightrope of life with steadiness and self-awareness.

Practice on the Mat

Brahmacharya is embodied by standing at the command center of our own power. We are the dispatchers, deciding when to send out more energy to poses and when to scale it back.

<u>Suggested One-Hour Asana Practice Considering Moderations and Variations</u>
A video to practice part of this sequence is available: courtneyseiberling.com/yoga

(All postures are held five breath cycles unless otherwise noted.)

Intention: *Give more energy to challenging postures. Sink into the relaxation of poses that require less. Back off poses that you don't have the energy for today.*

Hero on a Block (two minutes): *Survey the body and how you are feeling. Note your energy level. Do you need to push yourself today or take it easy?*

Yogi Bicycles (one minute, taking rest as needed)

Down Dog

Child's Pose (ten breath cycles, pausing at the top and bottom of each breath)

Plank (or stay in Child's Pose)

Cat/Cow (repeat five times)

Down Dog

Forward Fold

Sun A – arms up, Forward Fold, halfway lift, Forward Fold, arms up, hands in prayer at heart (repeat three times)

Chair

Sun B – Chair, Forward Fold, halfway lift, Forward Fold, Plank, Down Dog, Warrior One, Plank, Down Dog (repeat each side five times, taking Child's Pose as needed)

Chair Twist (each side)

Crescent (option to put knee down) to Crescent Twist (each side)

Wide-legged Forward Fold

Legs up the Wall or L

Superman (repeat three times)

Bridge (repeat three times) or Supported Bridge on Block

Reclined Twist (one minute each side)

Reclined Hamstring Stretch with Strap (each side)

Single or Reclined Pigeon (two minutes each side)
Happy Baby
Corpse (five to eight minutes)
Easy Seat: two-minute meditation

Consideration

Be aware of your energy and what you give it to. Throughout the week, make sure you offer the most energy to what matters!

Mantra

One thing at a time.

Personal Account

Like a lot of us, I tend to offer more of myself than I have to give. My default setting is to put others' needs first. I've poured my soul into friends' artistic endeavors and neglected my own. I've kept quiet in family relationships because I didn't want to upset the dynamics. I've dreamed my boyfriend's dreams instead of mine, and I've prioritized personal tasks in a pecking order that didn't reflect what was important to me, putting chores above my writing and treating fun as a reward instead of part of my daily routine. It's not that helping others or maintaining a clean house is wrong, but with only so many hours in a day, it's important to give ourselves to the things that matter most.

Of all the Yamas and Niyamas, Brahmacharya is the

principle I am the most focused on right now because it's the one that's challenging me. Today, I haven't done so well. All I wanted to do was write, and I'm just getting to it now at 9 p.m. Instead of writing earlier in the day, I busied myself with other things. I made items for my Etsy site, paid bills, cleaned, went to the grocery store, did research for my brother, read a friend's essay, scrolled social media, and met up with another friend to discuss an app she's developing. If I say I'm a writer, why was writing not a major part of my day?

Other essays in this book are about a specific situation I've resolved with a Yama or Niyama, but Brahmacharya is better shown through a collection of moments and how they fit together, so my application of this Yama spans many years.

***

Growing up, I was the good girl who was nice to everyone. I thought being liked was more important than anything, so I did everything I could to make sure people liked me. I worked extra hard to be an honors student. I volunteered at church. I overextended myself with activities and leadership positions at school and was a friend who would drop everything to listen. I didn't go to parties if there was a risk of getting in trouble. I didn't say anything that conflicted with what someone else thought. I did extra credit and exercised and wore makeup and cute outfits and decorated people's lockers on their birthdays. I smiled even if I was sad and laughed at jokes even if I found them offensive.

I fit myself into the mold other people's opinions made of me so I could feel secure. It was easier to be told who I was than to have to figure it out myself. I was friends with everyone not because I liked everyone but because it was easier to have friends than enemies. This was the reason why every year in high school, I was voted on the homecoming court. I didn't have a regular group of friends I ate lunch with and instead, floated from table to table. I hung out at both the soccer and football games. I was in the nerdy clubs and the cool ones. I auditioned for all the plays. I took music theory and AP courses and was the Class Secretary who chilled with the stoners. I dated the captain of the football team, a moody Bukowski fan, and a choir boy. I listened to Pearl Jam and pop music and was malleable enough to alter myself to be like whoever I was around.

But then, when I went off to college, no one knew who I was. The image I'd created was in a yearbook of the past. The girls on my dorm floor were shy or bold or strange but seemed to commit to whoever they were: a quiet concert violinist, a film buff, an Equestrian obsessed with *Winnie the Pooh*. My thing was that people liked me, but no one at school liked me yet, so I did the only thing I knew to do. I waited for other people to decide who I was. I was typecast as the ingénue in the college plays. I became known as the girl who baked cookies in the dorm because I did it once. I was told I hadn't lived at all by one of my acting professors, and I chose to believe it. I twisted through those four years, but I never developed myself enough at college to know who I was. This continued through my 20s. I was shy about my dreams. I let people take advantage of me. I completed a yoga teacher training because everyone told me I would be a good teacher but was intimidated by the instructors I loved and decided not to teach.

Then my 30s came. I wasn't as lost on who I was anymore, but I was working jobs that took too much of me. I was dating men who didn't understand me. I hadn't had success with my writing in the way I deserved. And then I realized something – this was all on me. It wasn't my boss's fault I left work exhausted; I was the one expecting too much of myself. I hadn't been picking the wrong men; I wasn't approaching relationships with my own self-worth. My writing hadn't taken off because I was hiding my gift on a computer instead of finding ways to share it.

I got so wrapped up in being nice and hardworking that I wasn't being very nice to myself. I hadn't spent enough time doing the things I actually wanted to do or going after what I desired. I created a dangerous thought and action pattern which became my routine and reality – to be busy instead of fulfilled, to work hard at work instead of on the book I wanted to write, to let fear take the lead in the dance of my life. I was giving my energy to anxiety and defeat instead of what I wanted and loved.

I decided to stop that story. I knew if I changed my story, it would change my life. I recognized myself as the author, and even if I don't have complete control over the way things go, I do have a say in what I spend my time on or at least what I do in my leisure. Now, instead of pushing myself to complete every task I'm assigned at work before going home, I leave on time and keep a pace where I can maintain my sanity. I speak up when I don't agree. I commit to the people I love, but I put myself first. I recognize if I want to be a writer, I must spend time writing, so I negotiated new hours with my employer to write in the morning before coming to work.

Realizing I decide who I am gave me the reins to a life I want. We all deserve the life we want. Don't waste precious time trying to make your father proud or allowing anyone else to steal your joy. It's a simple shift to own who you are and what you want to spend your time on. You can be angry. You can feel out of control. You can be a victim, or you can show up to what matters and deserves you. Yes, we all must do things we don't want to do. We have people who challenge us, but none of it needs to consume too much of our energy. Give yourself to you, and I'll keep giving myself to me.

Your Turn (to journal)

Write down everything you want to do this week. Make sure to include things that make you happy, like reading a book or spending time with a friend. Next, plan what you'll do when. See if you can let things fall away that don't really need to be done.

5 **APARIGRAHA** – LETTING GO

Aparigraha is the practice of non-attachment, of letting go and accepting what is. A friend and I both struggle with this concept and will half-jokingly, half-seriously text each other statements like:

Can't he just listen??
Why is it so hard to let go??!

It's hard to let go because it is, and yet all it takes is the decision to do so. Riding the waves of life instead of resisting them allows us to be in situations as they are without the stress of wanting them to be another way. This doesn't mean we give up or stop caring. It means we give in to what is true. We can't force our way back into someone's heart if they break up with us. We aren't returned an investment if we buy stock in a company that doesn't do well. It's understandable to be upset when things don't go as we hope, but when we linger in disappointment or attach to how we wanted something to be, we limit ourselves to what was and miss out on what is available now. There might be a better match we never would have met had our last partner not left or a lesson learned from a financial loss that influences the way we approach our next venture. Possibilities exist in the present, and it is up to us to live presently to make them possible.

Suffering is caused by our thoughts about a situation and not by the situation itself. Attaching to those thoughts turns them into stories, and stories become our perception of what is true, so we must be careful about the tales we tell ourselves! There could be a narrative that is no longer accurate or maybe never was. We have ideas about who we are, why things happen, and why other people do the things they do, but when we're able to let go of assumptions, we make space for the facts.

So how do we let go? The first step for me is to admit how I feel and to sit with that feeling. (*Why do I feel this way? What is this feeling about?*) The next step is to surrender to the truth which usually teaches me something I didn't know about myself. (*Oh! You're jealous! You haven't dealt with that thing from your past...*) Oftentimes, I'll learn I need to forgive another person, myself, or a situation. Aparigraha is the experience of forgiveness and surrender in order to get present. While forgiveness can seem difficult, it is also as easy as choosing to release and be at peace. When we forgive, nothing changes in the other person but something huge changes within us. The other person still did whatever they did and our acceptance of it doesn't give them permission to hurt us. We're already hurt. We don't punish someone by staying mad at them. We punish ourselves holding on to that hurt.

We must also extend forgiveness to ourselves and be careful not to get trapped in the past. Each day is a new opportunity to be in the life we want. To live with regret is to allow mistakes to stunt our growth. To be afraid of hurting others is to avoid connection altogether. When we own and accept what we've done and what's been done to us, the past stays in the past. When we don't, the past creeps into the present and dominates our current actions and decisions. Resentments can turn into toxins in the body and cause depression or sickness. Being gentle with ourselves and acknowledging feelings sets them free so we don't have to hold them.

Aparigraha loosens our grip on the future. So much of life is unpredictable and yet we try to plot it out to feel safe. We all know a person who has their whole life mapped out (maybe this person is you). They've decided what kind of spouse they want and how many children they will have. They've forecasted their career path and the amount of money they'll make and expect people will always do as they wish. It can be comforting to have plans, but stressful to count on them and devastating when life goes another way. I once had a smart and organized friend who wouldn't allow herself to retire until all her ducks were in a row and a very specific number was in her bank account. She was meticulous and patient and worked incessantly to put herself in this perfect place, and when she found herself there, she retired. Two months later, she died of an infection. It broke my heart to know life could be that unfair and reminded me how little control we have.

Like control, expectations can shade our experiences. It's one thing to be opportunistic and have goals but another to act entitled or hold ourselves to their fruition. When we make mental demands about how we want things to go, we are inflexible to how they may, and we set ourselves up for disappointment. We could miss an opportunity to learn something or obstruct a serendipitous direction. Antedating the future takes us out of the practice of living presently, and anticipating the actions of others impedes our ability to relate. When we expect a partner to read our mind, we assign him unrealistic, magical powers. If we put pressure on a friend to think like we do, we miss out on truly knowing her. Love requires us to accept and see people as they are and not grasp on to an image of how we want them to be. Making others responsible for our happiness places happiness outside ourselves. We already have everything we need, and Aparigraha asks us to remember it.

Another practice of Aparigraha is not to cling to material possessions or develop a false sense of ownership. Online shopping and retail therapy can be a quick fix of excitement but usually turn to buyer's remorse. The more we have, the more bills there are to pay, the more gadgets there are to maintain – items break, stain, or take up space in our homes after we become bored of them. We think we need more because advertising tells us we are not enough, but beauty creams, fancy cars, and workout programs rarely change anything if we aren't doing the work on the inside. The number of things we have and the status of their brands can make us feel important or give us a sense of identity but aren't as valuable as self-worth. Having stuff distracts us from just sitting with ourselves. Yes, sitting with ourselves can be scary and uncomfortable, but the more we are in the habit of it, the more connected we feel and the more authentically we live.

To choose Aparigraha is to choose freedom and to be content, whole, and unweighted by the decisions other people make. By doing so, we don't look to anyone or anything to determine our well-being. We witness what is true, and we accept what is real. We exist in the moment, withhold the past, and bravely welcome the unknowns of the future. We are empathetic, understanding, and trust life's lemons make delicious lemonade. By relinquishing control, we surrender to the Universe's plan and partner with it, our eyes wide-open with opportunity.

Practice on the Mat

Aparigraha is practiced by using the exhale to release. Stale air and tension fall away and make room for the present.

<u>Suggested One-Hour Asana Practice with a Focus on the Breath</u>
A video to practice part of this sequence is available: courtneyseiberling.com/yoga

(All postures are held five breath cycles unless otherwise noted.)

Intention: *Let go of tension in the body through exhalations.*
Easy Seat: Breath of Fire (three 30-second cycles)
Interlace fingers and send them over head
Seated Twist (each side)
Cat/Cow (repeat five times)

Child's Pose (five breath cycles, pausing at the top and bottom of each breath)
Down Dog
Forward Fold
Sun A – arms up, Forward Fold, halfway lift, Forward Fold, arms up, hands in prayer at heart (repeat three times)
Down Dog
Lizard (one minute each side)
Down Dog
Forward Fold
Chair
Chair Twist (each side)
Crescent to Crescent Twist (each side)
Wide-legged Forward Fold
Yogi Squat to Yogi Squat Twist (each side)
Legs up the Wall (two minutes)
Seated Wide-legged Forward Fold
Cobbler's
Head-to-Knee (each side)
Seated Forward Fold
Reclined Hamstring Stretch with Strap (each side)
Happy Baby
Reclined or Single Pigeon (two minutes each side)
Reclined Twist (each side)
Corpse (five to eight minutes)
Easy Seat: three-minute meditation

Consideration

Can you let go of your expectations and be with others as they are?

Mantra

Give up. Give in. Let go.

Personal Account

When I was in my 20s and living in New York City, I reconnected with a man I knew from college who played in a band in Los Angeles. I heard a song he wrote, reached out to him, and a flurry of communication erupted between us. He was funny, smart, deep…everything I thought I wanted in a partner, and I saw something in him I hadn't seen before: a future. We fell fast and hard in love swapping books and tunes, thoughts and dreams. He was the first person to hold my interest, and he became more interesting to me with time. I couldn't imagine my life without him now that he was in it, so I left the city I loved and moved 3,000 miles west.

Our bond was everything I hoped for: epic admiration, long talks, grand adventures, and I never saw it ending like I had in my other relationships. But then, after three and a half wonderful years together, he left me without a warning. I came home from work one day and found him crying on our couch. I assumed something was wrong with his father, who was an alcoholic, and rushed to him, but he stopped me and said, "I'm leaving you for S."

S. was our mutual friend and former roommate who'd been dating our other friend and former roommate for several years. I thought it was a joke. My boyfriend and I had just moved into our own place, and he'd written me a long letter saying how happy he was. It couldn't be true, I decided, as I unpacked the groceries for the dinner I was still planning to make. In the midst of chopping lettuce, my boyfriend's phone rang, and he took the call outside. It was S. I recognized her ringtone. I put down the knife and went to the window, watching my boyfriend pace the patio. *What was he saying that he couldn't say in front of me? How could he not look up to consider me as he considered another life?* After hanging up, my boyfriend walked toward the gate and then out of it. I heard his car start and rattle off, and then I heard nothing but the loudest silence. I couldn't believe this was happening, that a person who loved me loved someone else enough to leave me.

There were so many logistics. I told our new landlords we needed to break the lease. I looked for a new place to live that I could afford on my own, and I packed up the things I'd just unpacked. As I unhooked frames from the wall, I wondered, *What do you do with photographs that tell the story of a life you thought you'd have?* I cancelled the surprise 30th birthday party I'd been planning for my boyfriend and took care of his dog who kept peeing in the house and running away. I comforted our friends who were upset about the breakup and recounted the story enough times until it began to feel true. I became obsessed with the thought of my boyfriend having hot, new sex with someone who I had trusted. It was awful. More awful than it sounds. I didn't sleep for weeks. I couldn't eat. I looked terrible. I felt worse. For the first time in my life, I was experiencing real heartbreak.

A year went by, and I still didn't have any closure. I held on to the thought that my funny, smart, and deep man would show up one day after he realized he'd made a mistake and demand I take him back. I continued to work on the documentary I was making about his band so I could listen to his jokes and hear songs he'd written. Because we shared so many friends, I occasionally saw him and S. at parties and showers, and he was always there in the tension of my right hip during my yoga practice. I longed for him and begged the Universe to return him back to me because that is where he belonged.

Then came the two-year mark of our separation, and he still hadn't come back. He got engaged to S. He married her. I sat at my computer on the night of their wedding, stalking our shared friends' Facebook pages for pictures of the event as it was happening in real time. I sobbed with jealousy as I stared at the stills. They looked the happiest I'd ever seen either of them. Another year went by, and they stayed married. I fantasized about driving to their house with a box of old photographs and setting fire to it on the front lawn. Then another year passed, and they got pregnant. By this time, I'd dated other people and was with a man who loved me dearly. We bought a house and moved in, and you may think this is the part where I say I forgave my ex-boyfriend, but it isn't. Intellectually, I knew I was better off, but forgiving my ex made it seem like what he had done was okay, and it wasn't.

After I moved into that house with the man who loved me dearly, a different man walked into my yoga class and stopped my heart. We chatted after class and after only a few minutes, he asked me out. I told him I had a boyfriend but we could be friends, and we agreed to meet for coffee a few days later. Coffee turned into a walk in the park and then a long cry in my car. I knew I could never see him again. I went home and told my boyfriend what had happened. I meant it to be a conversation about choice and commitment, but it emitted an awful series of misunderstandings, and I became so frustrated with the assumptions and accusations my boyfriend was making that I left him the following week. In almost an instant, I saw how little he worked to understand me and my complexities, how he wouldn't hear the truth. I thought of my ex-boyfriend's journey with S. and the time I'd found him crying on the couch – that there was nothing he could have said or done to make it right. He knew in his gut I wasn't the one, and I knew the man I was living with in this beautiful house wasn't mine either. Even though the situations weren't the same, the outcome was: someone had to leave a person they loved because they knew a different life would be better. And suddenly, instead of my ex being a monster, he became a person. And instead of feeling like a monster, I saw myself as a person who had to make a really difficult decision and did.

A month after I left the house and my boyfriend, I wrote my ex and S. I'd wanted to write this letter for years, but it had always felt disingenuous. I wrote the letter for me, saying I forgave them, acknowledging how hard it must have been to make the decision they did, and I understood why. I wished them happiness on the anticipated arrival of their child, and I meant every word. As I put the letter in the blue metal box, the tension in my right hip lessened. I felt lighter than I had in god knows how long. I was truly okay.

A few weeks later, I went to a baby shower, aware that my ex and S. were also invited. Even though I wasn't as nervous as I usually was when I had to see them, I still didn't want to go. I arrived late, staying on the perimeter of the guests, finding my way through the friends I knew. I could see S. in my periphery, aware it would only be moments before I'd have to address her. Standing near the gift table, alone in all her beautiful mama-to-be-ness, I decided to make the move. I walked to the table, opened my heart, and put her in my arms, feeling her stomach full of the love she made to the man I once thought was my forever person. But he was her forever person. We talked. We cried. We laughed. My ex came over, and we did it all over again. Then, he and S. handed me letters they wrote in response to mine — one from each of them. I hadn't expected it, thanked them, and went home.

The next morning, I tucked the letters into my back pocket and hiked up a mountain near my apartment. When I reached the top, I found a ledge to sit on and read words of pain and guilt. This whole time, I thought my ex and S. hadn't thought of me at all, but I learned they still carried me with them. They hadn't let go either. As I read the people I once knew and loved, I could feel them knowing and loving me again. They were releasing me just as I had released them.

Sometimes when we really love someone, we must let them go, especially if they head in direction we cannot follow.

Your Turn (to journal)

What is taking up your headspace in an unproductive way? Is it something or someone from the past? What would your life look like if you weren't thinking about it?

THE **NIYAMAS** – HOW TO CARE FOR YOURSELF

The Niyamas are five practices from the Yoga Sutras that suggest how to care for yourself. Keeping things neat and tidy puts the mind at ease. Being content grounds us in reality. Allowing feelings to be felt helps us heal. Developing self-awareness shows us what's important so we can work hard to go after what we want. Life is incessantly more meaningful when we open to the wonder around us and celebrate it.

Practicing the Niyamas is like a spa day for the soul. When we take time to slow down, know ourselves, and notice beauty, we live more fully and feel more connected.

6 **SAUCHA** – ORDER

Saucha, order, is the act of keeping things clean and uncluttered. When physical spaces are neat, the mind can focus. The body more easily processes food if it is clear of toxins. While the simplest of the Yamas and Niyamas to understand, Saucha can be difficult to implement. As busy people, obsessed with accomplishments and productivity, we push ourselves to do and be more. Our homes, studios, and offices are often messy reflections of the fast pace we keep to maintain a go-go-go lifestyle, and residing in chaotic spaces encourages the mind to race, making life feel more overwhelming than it already is.

We practice Saucha by picking up after ourselves and making sure areas are clean and organized. Consider starting with one space like your car. Bring in your traveler's mug when you finish your coffee. Throw away food wrappers after you eat. Organize papers in your glove box and only leave items in your console that you need. Keep spare change in a container and your sunglasses in a designated area where they can be easily located. Maintaining order in your car can steady the mind so you're more focused and calm when you reach your destination. If you notice results, try it at home. Put things away when you are finished with them and wash dishes after dinner instead of leaving pots and plates in the sink. Dust regularly and keep floors and counters clean. Donate items you don't use or clothes you don't wear so your closet and living spaces are more spacious. Your head and heart will feel more spacious, too.

Next, be aware of what you put in your body and how you feel afterwards. Do you notice when you eat rich foods, you feel sluggish? Or when you have that extra glass of wine, you wake up the next day an hour later than you wanted? Drink more water and less caffeine. Eat more fruits and vegetables than meat, flour, and refined sugar. Practice yoga or take a walk after work to unclutter your mind from the day. Acknowledge emotions as they're felt so they can flow and not become lodged in the body. Take a nap or a painting class on a free afternoon instead of attacking the next item on your to-do list. There are so many small ways to make space, and our choices leave us clean and clear or lethargic and heavy.

Saucha can also be applied to our relationships. The people we spend time with either encourage us to feel light and optimistic or weigh us down with negativity and drama. We easily absorb the stress of others. Removing those who disturb our true, calm nature from our contact lists and setting boundaries with challenging people at work ensures our joy isn't disrupted. While it can be uncomfortable to limit or end relationships entirely, it creates room for those who inspire and energize us.

Even when we spend time with good people, we can overextend and give more of ourselves than we have to offer. Practicing Saucha in our friendships means we make plans with others when we can be present. Sometimes, we need time alone to journal, read, or exercise to recharge and balance our spirit. Schedule solo dates before social ones, and treat yourself with the same love and care you afford friends and family.

Saucha makes room for the present. Notice your breath and how it releases stress and brings you into the here and now. Whenever you remember, take a breath to clear space in your body and mind.

Practice on the Mat

Yoga is detoxifying — a steam clean for the system. Saucha uses breath and movement to release toxins, old thought patterns, and tension.

<u>Suggested One-Hour Asana Practice with an Emphasis on Twists</u>
A video to practice part of this sequence is available: courtneyseiberling.com/yoga

(All postures are held five breath cycles unless otherwise noted.)

Intention: *Can you create space in your body with the breath?*
Easy Seat: two-minute meditation focusing on the breath
Breath of Fire (three 30-second cycles)
Seated Twist (each side)

Cat/Cow
Sunbird – twist back and grab foot (each side)
Down Dog
Down Dog Twist (each side)
Sun A – arms up, Forward Fold, halfway lift, Forward Fold, arms up, hands in prayer at heart (repeat three times)
Down Dog to Tiger to knee opposite elbow to One-legged Down Dog (each side)
Crescent to Crescent Twist (each side)
Chair to Chair Twist (each side)
Sun A – arms up, Forward Fold, halfway lift, Forward Fold, arms up, hands in prayer at heart
Crescent Twist (each side)
Wide-legged Forward Fold Twist (each side)
Tree (knee in to hip height and twist, each side)
Legs up the Wall (two minutes)
Cobbler's
Head-to-Knee (each side)
Cow Face with Shoulder Opener (each side)
Reclined Hamstring Stretch with Strap (each side)
Reclined Pigeon (two minutes each side)
Reclined Cow Face (one minute each side)
Reclined Twist (each side)
Corpse (five to eight minutes)

Consideration

Can you clean out one space that you use frequently – a drawer, your car, a closet?

Can you be conscious of what you eat and drink and notice how you feel after you do?

Mantra

Clean and clear.

Personal Account

I started to keep a friend at an arm's length when I realized she was taking advantage of my kindness. Let's call her Sarah. Sarah was the friend I had over for dinner a lot who never cooked for me and expected me to pay when we went out for coffee or a drink because she couldn't hold down a job. She always had car trouble, always dominated conversations with her relationship drama, and she couldn't seem to get herself on her own two feet. I felt like I was always holding her up, but she was charismatic and fun, and I cared about her, so I kept showing up in a big way. I figured she was going through a hard time and told myself she needed extra support now and our relationship would become balanced when she got to the other side.

Sarah was in an unhealthy relationship and lived with a boyfriend who pressured her to do cocaine every Friday night. She hated this ritual because she didn't like who he became when he used the drug, and her Saturdays were spent recovering from the prior evening's shenanigans. The pattern kept repeating. On Mondays, I would receive a call and listen to her cry about how they'd done it again. I encouraged her to tell him she wanted to stop, but the following week, she'd call again, and we'd have the same conversation. After months and months, she got up the courage to leave. I was relieved but also scared for her. She didn't have any money saved, and she needed a place to go. She had financially tapped out her dad, so I told her she could stay with me until she figured it out. At the time, I was living in a studio and going through a hard period of my own.

Sarah showed up to my place with a few bags and her cat. I didn't have the heart to tell her how horribly allergic I was, so I welcomed them both inside and decided I'd sniffle my way through it. While I was at work, Sarah ate my food. She broke dishes. The contents of her suitcase spilled over my living area so the apartment appeared more cramped and small than it was, but I reminded myself of how overwhelmed she must be and didn't criticize her. I made dinner for us, and we drank wine and had lovely conversations.

A week into her stay, Sarah went to visit a friend in Northern California and sent me a text from the road saying she'd be gone a few days and wanted to know if I'd look after her cat. I thought it was strange to leave without asking first, but I was grateful to have a little time to myself again, so I said it wasn't a problem. Only, it was a problem. The cat rubbed himself on my face while I slept, and I had trouble breathing. He scratched at the walls and furniture and went to the bathroom in the corners of my apartment. I was miserable and mad at myself for not telling my friend to find another place for him while she was gone and communicated that she had to come back for the cat and find another place to stay. I felt horrible for retracting what I offered, but my decision to let her stay had put me in a vulnerable situation. I should have set parameters that honored both her needs and mine, and I hadn't.

This is what we call boundaries. Boundaries are the way to establish what you can and can't accept from people.

Because my inclination is to give and give, Saucha is a practice I remind myself of a lot. I came up against it recently when a friend asked to borrow my studio for a photo shoot. I rent it for income, so I had to block it off for a couple days to accommodate her and take a small, financial loss. My friend didn't offer compensation, but I didn't mind because I like to support friends' creative endeavors, and this was a way I could. My friend made a mess of the studio and didn't help me clean up. She used my food and wine for some of her shots and didn't restock my fridge or reimburse me. I'd given up a day of working on my own projects to grocery shop, make lunch for her crew, and schlep props in and out of the space, and I felt underappreciated and offended until I realized I hadn't set boundaries with her. I kept offering more of myself with a smile. I should have started our initial conversation, "Yes, you can use the studio, BUT please make sure to…" instead of saying, "Yes, whatever you need." It was another reminder to be upfront and clear about what I expect from someone else so there is an understanding of what will be given and what will be received.

I have a deep respect and appreciation for those who have set boundaries with me so I know what the confines of the relationship are. Ex-boyfriends have distanced or changed the intimacy or frequency of our communication, and it's created healthier, more defined relationships. Some have removed me from their lives completely, but that clearing of the past is sometimes necessary to live in the present. We must know ourselves, what we want and need, and what conflicts with it. When we own our limitations and desires and can communicate it clearly, we establish a clean and balanced existence with others.

Your Turn (to journal)

Where do you need to establish boundaries or set limits?

7 **SANTOSHA** – CONTENTMENT

Santosha translates as contentment. To be content, we must trust, have patience, and be present with whatever is happening whether we like it or not. Rather than think, *I'll be okay WHEN...* we make the decision to be okay NOW and to exist in the moment that is. Growing up, my father said I got to choose whether or not I was going to have a good day or a bad day, and it was dependent on how I saw and handled situations. I could get mad and fight back, or I could surrender to what was happening and be at peace. Whenever I picked the latter, I had a good day even if it didn't go according to plan. Without knowing it then, my father was teaching me the practice of Santosha.

Santosha allows us to be with things as they are without wishing circumstances to be different. This is not passive behavior but proactive in that it enables our perception to influence perspective. Experiences are all how we see them. We can witness things as unfair and happening *to* us, or we can take the cards we are dealt and be a part of the game.

We can dislike the outcome of something and still find our place in it. We can stay true to who we are as we hear other viewpoints. Differences may even strengthen our commitment to what we believe or open our minds to what we hadn't considered. Instead of playing the victim when something bad happens, we can ask, *What is this situation here to teach me*? Oftentimes there is a lesson, and yet sometimes there isn't. Terrible things can happen for little reason, but contentment keeps us grounded so we can move through tough times with fortitude and grace.

Santosha places us in the eye of the storm without reaction. Instead of fighting and flailing, we are supple and know the storm will pass. Life is unpredictable and when we acknowledge it, we are better equipped to move into new phases calm and ready. If nothing ever tested us, we would never grow. Each push makes us more experienced. Every stress builds character. When we resist change, we diminish the opportunities of the present. We have a choice to be bitter and guarded or understanding and available. We can open our hearts and forgive or we can close them off and refuse to forget. What kind of person do you want to be? The one who shuts down or the one who confides in the wild ride of life, understanding it to be full of humility, humor, disappointment, and possibility? Contentment is the seat belt that keeps us safe by keeping us centered.

Contentment shouldn't be confused with happiness. We can be content but not happy. When facing difficulty, contentment stops us from expending energy wanting it to be another way. The only way it can be is the way it is, and Santosha holds us in that veracity.

Another aspect of contentment is to love and accept

ourselves for who we are and not wish others to think or act differently than they do. I like to think everyone is doing their best with the tools they have and that some of us have better toolboxes than others. Acceptance of ourselves and others is the greatest thing we can offer our relationships so they can be loving and empathetic.

A practice of contentment is one in which we admit reality and stop escaping to alternative outcomes. We put faith in the ebb and flow of things and trust in the Universe, other people, and ourselves. We stay grounded in the mantra *Life isn't always fair*, yet treat situations fairly. By making the choice to be okay, we ARE okay.

Practice on the Mat

On the mat, Santosha is a practice of managing expectations. Take rest when needed and be with the body as it is today.

<u>Suggested One-Hour Balancing Asana Practice</u>
A video to practice part of this sequence is available: courtneyseiberling.com/yoga

(All postures are held five breath cycles unless otherwise noted.)

Intention: *Own your level of practice. Honor where you are and accept your limitations.*
Easy Seat: *Close your eyes. How are you feeling? Really breathe into that feeling and claim it, whether you want to be feeling that way or not.*

Mountain Pose with hands in prayer at heart: *Close your eyes and survey your energy level. Know where you are.*
Forward Fold – clasp hands or a strap and send arms up and overhead
Balance on toes (repeat three times)
Standing Split with hands on Blocks (each side)
Cross at the ankles, halfway lift, Forward Fold with hands on Blocks (each side)
Sun A – arms up, Forward Fold, halfway lift, Forward Fold, arms up, hands in prayer at heart (repeat five times)
Plank to Forearm Plank (repeat three times)
Dolphin (one minute)
Child's Pose
Plank
Side Plank (each side)
Warrior Two (10 breath cycles) to Side Angle to Triangle to Half Moon to Forward Fold (each side)
Wide-legged Forward Fold
Standing Pigeon to Tree to Eagle (each side)
Legs up the Wall (two minutes)
Camel at the Wall (repeat two times)
Cobra (repeat three times)
Sphinx (take neck rolls each way)
Superman
Bridge (repeat three times)
Reclined Twist (each side)
Reclined Cow Face (two minutes each side)
Happy Baby
Corpse (five to eight minutes)

Consideration

Can you catch yourself when you think, *I'll be okay when...* and choose to be okay now?

Mantra

Trust it's okay.

Personal Account

Early in my professional life, I worked an entry-level position in Communications. I had a thoughtful boss who I respected for her forward-looking, clear direction, and she didn't push me too hard. She understood the job was just a job for me, and my ambitions were in the arts. I did good work when I was in the office but didn't do anything beyond my position or pay grade. I put in my eight hours, took lunch, and did what was asked of me at a pace I found reasonable. When I left, I didn't check email or think about work so I could focus on my own interests.

But then something sneaky happened. I got interested in the work. My boss and I were building a brand together, telling stories about women who mattered and did incredible things in the world, and I enjoyed writing about them. Social media was new and exploding, and online publications were a necessary addition to print materials. There was suddenly so much more to do, and my boss was working all the time, but I still left at the end of my eight-hour shift. It made me feel guilty, and even though I cared more, it wasn't enough to make me stay late.

The biggest challenge in our four years together was marketing a centennial celebration. It just about killed us, but my boss and I became stronger as a team, and she did a fantastic job leading the business into its next century. At the culminating gala, we were tired and proud, and it wasn't long after the event that my boss took another job at another non-profit. It was a financial bump for her, and she was ready for a new challenge. I was sad to see her go because she had become a dear friend, but I was happy she was taking the next step in her professional development.

I wasn't eligible or interested in being promoted and knew my organization would hire someone who I would have to work with intimately. I expected the new director would value my institutional knowledge and the longevity I had with the organization. I suspected we would become friends because this always happened with my managers. I consider myself an open, amicable person, and I was excited about the potential of learning from another professional.

My boss's replacement was a friendly, upbeat woman who was easy-going and fun. I was smitten. We chatted about the best places in the area for lunch, and she took my recommendations. She was interested in learning about my artistic ambitions, and I was encouraged to assume she would become my friend and value my work parameters. I kept at the easy pace I was used to and was forward about the particulars of our brand. After a few months, my new boss and I were in the weeds with summer projects. She had less initial vision than my former boss and gave me flexibility to run with ideas on my own. Initially, it was liberating, but then it became daunting. I craved direction and specifics of what she was looking for and wished she'd be as clear as the previous director.

To accommodate the new working style, I stayed late a couple nights a week to work on projects which escalated to almost every night. I neglected my own artistic endeavors and skipped my workouts. This new, work-centered life was frustrating, foreign, and seemed endless. One morning, after spending hours the night before developing a concept for a pamphlet, my new boss offered ambiguous feedback.

"Maybe it should have more pizazz!" she suggested. "What if it took a more direct approach?"

I was like...*huh*?! and went back to my computer to figure out what "pizazz" looked like for the rest of the day.

This continued with other projects. It was a lot of trial and error, and I came home most nights crying to my poor boyfriend about how unclear and lax my boss was – that she didn't care about the brand my former boss and I had methodically shaped. My boyfriend heard my hysterical frustration more times than I'd like to admit, and after many patient nights listening to me blubber into my wine glass, he told me there was no need to be so wrecked about it, and I should change my attitude. I knew he was right. I needed to stop taking work home with me.

But instead of shifting my attitude about work, I decided the thing that needed changing was my boss. I scheduled a meeting to explain how hard it was to work with her. I was professional, yet hinted at her confusing directional style. I asked if she could be clearer about what she wanted from the beginning and said it would make things easier for us both. I expressed concern over the design going in a whole other direction; the new, casual voice of our marketing materials didn't sound like us; and we were straying from our font and style guide. (These meetings happened more than once.) She kindly listened but still pushed us in a new direction. My boss's boss loved what we were up to, and I felt more and more alone as I continued to protest my loyalty to what had been. We finished projects, but there were many more twists and turns than I was used to making before we landed somewhere. My new boss kept nudging us farther away from the voice, look, and feel of the past until what I'd worked so hard to protect was almost unrecognizable. After about a year and a half of resisting her and the work, I gave my notice.

At my next job, my boss was charismatic, smart, and capable. I liked him right away. Even though he was new to the institution, he appeared expedient in his position. We laughed easily, and he supported my ambitions outside of work. But after a few months, I realized I was in over my head. There was so much work to do and more emails than I could answer in a day. I stayed late and worked through lunch and didn't socialize with my colleagues, but the work still piled up and never seemed to be done. I was exhausted and irritable, and when I talked to my boss about it, he told me to stop working so much.

"But then the work won't get done!" I objected.

He shrugged his shoulders casually and said something like, "It's not worth breaking yourself over," before going home to his family.

Like my former boss, my new one provided little direction and trusted me to do my work. He didn't know the ins and outs of my job, and I felt buried in the details. He didn't sweat the small stuff or address problems until they were *really* problems. My late nights became later and the crying to my boyfriend reemerged. Frustrated, I swore if my boss would just care more and step it up, I wouldn't have to be so miserable and overwhelmed. It was just as it had been with my last boss, and I realized the common denominator in both situations was not them but me.

What was *I* doing wrong? Why was I so stressed and frustrated with people? Then something knocked me over the head. This had come up with my Mom, too. Whenever we didn't see eye to eye, I wanted her to be and act other than she was being and acting. She called me out on it one day.

"You're trying to change me," she said.

And I was. This is exactly what I was doing with my last two bosses. I wanted them to value what I valued in the way I valued it. I wanted them to focus on the things I focused on and put their own visions and work styles aside. Perhaps the new direction my former boss took wasn't the wrong direction, just different. Maybe my new boss was onto something about not getting swept up in the day-to-day details and dramas. They were each smart and respected employees of their institution, and the only person who wasn't respecting them was me.

I needed to put aside my own agenda and see what my boss's was. I'd missed that opportunity with the previous one, but I could start with him. Instead of obsessing about all the things he wasn't doing, I noticed what he was. And you know what? He was doing a lot. I began to admire his assets and didn't hold him liable for any shortcomings. Instead of trying to make him be the boss I wanted, I let him be the boss he was. Rather than wish he'd care more about the minutia, I valued his temperate reactions and humor. Instead of being annoyed when he didn't remember something, I was pleased at how quickly he problem-solved.

This shift was a remarkable change in how I felt at work and most importantly, what I stopped taking home with me. Instead of crying and complaining, I acknowledged what my boss offered: priorities, perspective, and balance; the value of taking things less seriously and forcefully; and the benefit of meeting people where they are.

****

Bringing contentment into my personal and professional relationships has limited my demands on them and transformed my interactions. I don't carry so many presumptions, and I'm able to see people's good qualities over their bad. Rather than expect my friends to support me through every bad day I have, I appreciate whenever they check in with me. Instead of staying home and dreaming up the perfect guy who checks off all my boxes, I opened myself to other possibilities and met a man at a coffee shop who was not what I expected and everything I didn't know I needed. Life is abundant and surprising when we stop limiting how we think it should be and allow it to be as it is.

Your Turn (to journal)

Think of a time when you fought. What would have been the outcome if you stopped fighting and started listening?

8 **TAPAS** – DISCIPLINE AND DISCOMFORT

Tapas is a Niyama with two schools of thought. Commonly referred to as "burning enthusiasm," Tapas is first a discipline practice, the act of taking interest in something and pursuing it with fervor. Fueling the fire of our passions ignites us with purpose so we feel connected to what we are doing. The second practice of Tapas allows discomfort to be a part of life. Instead of brushing feelings under the rug, we let ourselves stew in them so we can process and move through emotion.

Let's investigate the discipline practice of Tapas first. If yoga means union, then our most balanced, whole self is the one in which we allow ourselves to be who we are, doing what we love. When we are not in this alignment, we suffer and feel lost, bored, or depressed. If you don't know what you love, want to study, or what job or hobbies to pursue, pay attention to what interests and excites you, and the answers are often there. Tapas can be a guide to discover passion and develop a commitment to it. It's important to be present and stay open to what you're curious about now, not what you've been interested in before. What presents itself might be a surprise. It may not be logical, linear, or have any monetary benefit, but it's worth staying to explore. Give yourself fully to this hobby or interest. Learn the nuts and bolts. What you put your energy into will grow and with more time comes more skill. Through a disciplined practice, tasks prioritize themselves, and you'll feel less overwhelmed by the things that don't matter and more energized by the things that do.

It takes a while to get good at something, but sticking with it refines our skills. Mastery is not the result of a fast-track of luck but a long ride of perseverance. An athlete isn't only gifted with skill; he spends hours performing drills and improving his footwork. A songwriter doesn't sit down to write a song and play the finished one we hear on the radio; she starts with a phrase and builds on it. An artist might spend months on a painting and then scrap it altogether. A filmmaker shoots plenty of footage that is never seen. Most of what's created is never experienced by an audience, but the magic is in the doing, in developing a relationship with a skill. Entrepreneurs and engineers work extensively behind the scenes to shape a business platform or product – some flop, others take off, yet much is gained either way. A CEO rarely starts at the head of a company nor does a celebrity rise to overnight stardom even if it appears that way. In Tapas, success isn't measured by recognition but in the dedication to the process. The work becomes more satisfying than the outcome. Wonder awakens a sense of purpose, and meaning arises from commitment.

Tapas is a wonderful relational practice as well. When we show up fully to the people we care about and are present in our interactions, our relationships flourish. We often receive back the same respect, attention, and care we give as we engage and commit to others – assumptions, selfishness, jealousy, and other relationship-killers fall away. A husband's devotion is experienced as he listens to his spouse's concerns over dinner. A mother's dedication keeps her engaged in the challenge of breastfeeding. A friend stands by her girlfriend even if she doesn't understand or agree with her choices. Tapas fires up our accountability to other people and makes us superheroes to those we love.

But Tapas isn't only about the passions we seek. It's about the ones that seek us – the fires that simmer from within. In addition to a discipline practice, Tapas is also a way to let emotions burn by allowing them to be fully felt. Taking interest in our pain makes us a part of the experience and not separate from it. Instead of distracting ourselves from how we feel with work or drinking, we lean into suffering to process and move through it so we don't carry residual trauma or resentment. We comfort sadness and anger when we admit them. We step through darkness to find light. It can be hard, unfun work to embrace the disruptions of life and stay in the heat of discomfort, but when we do, we release what has happened and are free to be with what is.

Practice on the Mat

A regular fitness practice builds resilience in the muscles and develops Tapas, discipline. As the layers of the body burn and release toxins, mental strength kicks in when we want to give up.

<u>Suggested One-Hour Asana Practice with Long Holds</u>
A video to practice part of this sequence is available: courtneyseiberling.com/yoga

(All postures are held seven breath cycles unless otherwise noted.)

Intention: *Take interest in every pose. Lean into any discomfort and stay (unless there is sharp pain).*
Reclined Bound Angle with Blocks under knees
Leg Lowers (support low back with tops of hands underneath hip bone, hover feet one inch from floor, then lift feet above hips; repeat 10 times)
Hug knees to chest, roll knees clockwise and counterclockwise; roll up to stand
Mountain Pose
Sun A – arms up, Forward Fold, halfway lift, Forward Fold, arms up, hands in prayer at heart (repeat three times)
Sun B – Chair, Forward Fold, halfway lift, Forward Fold, Plank, Down Dog, Warrior One, Plank, Down Dog (repeat each side three times)
Child's Pose
Down Dog
Tiger to knee opposite elbow to One-legged Down Dog (repeat each side three times)
Warrior One (10 breath cycles) to Humble Warrior to Pyramid to Down Dog (each side)
Warrior Two to Side Angle to Triangle to Down Dog (each side)
Wide-Legged Forward Fold
Chair Twist (each side)
Eagle (each side)
Handstand or Legs up the Wall (two minutes)

Bridge or Wheel (repeat five times)
Reclined Twist (each side)
Single or Reclined Pigeon (two minutes each side)
Happy Baby
Cobbler's
Seated Wide-Legged Forward Fold
Head-to-Knee (each side)
Seated Forward Fold
Corpse (five to eight minutes)

Consideration

Can you be more engaged in what you are doing, especially when it is something you are passionate about?

Mantra

Stay. Experience. Learn.

Personal Account

When I was 23, I was raped. It happened in a high-rise apartment building in a safe and residential New York City neighborhood by a man who was a regular at the restaurant where I worked. I wasn't attracted to him or interested in dating, but he was pushy and potently charming and kept asking me to go out with him until I said I would. We met at a burrito place, and I was surprised to like his company enough to agree to see him again.

The thing no one tells you about sexual assault is that it

usually happens with someone you know, not when a stranger jumps out from behind a bush late at night and forces himself on you. I imagined it would be the latter by the way I was prepped during college orientation. A staff member handed me a branded whistle and said I should blow hard and kick a guy in the balls or pee on myself if someone tried something. But I didn't have a whistle when it happened to me, and the thought of kicking the guy in the balls or peeing on myself didn't cross my mind. I was on a date.

My restaurant pursuer suggested I come to his place for a drink before we went out that second time. I felt like I knew him well enough to go to his apartment. I'd seen him a dozen or so times at the restaurant, we'd been out once before, and I was flattered he wanted to show me where he lived. I arrived at our agreed time of 7 p.m., and the doorman sent me up. My date opened the door, splashed in designer cologne and fashioned neatly. I was excited for our evening together. I followed him into the kitchen where he was making drinks: gin, I remember every time I smell gin. Music played. Billy Joel or something that sounded like Billy Joel. My pursuer offered me one of the concoctions he'd made, took the other for himself, and directed me into the living room. We talked cozily on the couch until the album finished about I don't know what. We had nothing in common except the restaurant where we met. About three fourths of the way into my drink, something started to feel wrong. It became hard to focus, and the room got fuzzy. I knew alcohol hit hard on an empty stomach, but this was something else.

Not wanting to make a scene, I suggested we head to dinner, and he brushed it off as the city sounds below became long and slow. I kept sipping the drink to be polite, trying to concentrate on whatever it was he was saying, but words were blending together like an abstract painting. I placed my attention on one thing at a time to steady myself: the lift of my finger; setting down the glass; nodding my head to imply I was listening. The last thing I remember was falling off the couch and laughing uncomfortably and then waking up on the bed naked with him above me, his forehead wet with sweat and elation, and not being able to get up or say no.

I must have fallen into a deep sleep that lasted the duration of the night, because the next thing I recall was a window washer squeegeeing the glass bordering the bed as the sun lifted a new day. The bright light was harsh on the scene: Him. Me. Messy sheets around our ankles. I slid from them and collected my clothes, leaving as quietly as I could so as not to wake him. The air outside hit my cheeks hard, and I cried. My body was heavy. My heart packed with shame. *How did I let this happen?* I thought, as I walked the gray streets and swore I'd tell no one how drunk or dumb I'd been.

It didn't even cross my mind I'd been assaulted, and it wasn't until a year later, watching television, when I realized what had happened. A character at a party had something slipped into her drink and as the room slowed and spun from her POV, it became my own in the high-rise building on that second date. As I witnessed the TV character fall to the floor, I remembered how it had been to lose my inhibitions. I watched in horror as a guy lifted up the character, took her into a room, and put himself inside her while she lay open and limp on a bed. The next morning, her pee smelled weird like mine had. But the difference between the character and me was she understood what happened to her right away, and I was only becoming aware of it now. She wanted revenge. I was embarrassed.

Trauma shielded my impulse to act or unravel in the aftermath. I convinced myself I'd gotten drunk even though I only had one drink (that I remember). I blamed myself for going to someone's apartment I barely knew, for not saying something was wrong when I felt it was wrong. After realizing I'd been the victim of a horrific incident, I was ashamed for not having reported it. My lack of action could have resulted in my pursuer doing what he did to me to other women. I tried to get up the nerve to call the police, but I only had a blanched memory of what happened, and I doubted my story. As more time passed, I remembered less. I forgot what street he lived on and where he worked, his physical features dim. I tried to find him on Facebook, but the only person with his name was a woman.

As I externalized what happened by trying to act and save others, I realized the person who needed saving was myself. This was the beginning of my healing: admitting I'd been raped, that it wasn't my fault, and knowing I had to do the work to heal. The next step was to sit in the discomfort, the Tapas, and process the experience. It was like being stuck in a coat with a broken zipper. My body felt soiled, tampered with, discharged, like it wasn't mine anymore. I wanted to run from my feelings but knew the only way out of the situation was through it, and I needed to reclaim my body. For six months, I practiced yoga every day. I stood on my mat or laid on it when that was all I could do, and I committed to the gentle, agonizing work. I watched my thigh shake in Warrior One. I found stillness and strength in

Warrior Two. I fell. I flowed. I breathed. I stayed when it was uncomfortable, and I released wherever and whenever I could. Eventually, I felt an arm again and then a leg and then how they were connected to my shoulder and hip. As I softened, my body came back to me and was mine again.

***

A practice of Tapas means we stay. We experience the pain, uneasiness, or embarrassment to move beyond it. This is also the practice I apply when I sit down to write. I'll doubt myself. Some mornings, I rewrite sentences or have less of them than when I began, but I trust and know the only way projects come into being is through commitment, hard work, and going through the (not so) fun house of the process. On the other side is a book or a strengthened part of ourselves that has faced what we needed to: the darkness, our shadows, the parts of others we don't want to believe are possible. But when we do, things begin to feel possible again.

Your Turn (to journal)

What are you sweeping under the rug? Can you write about it for 10 minutes and get to know it?

9 **SVADHYAYA** – SELF-STUDY

One of the greatest things we can do for our emotional and mental well-being is to practice *Svadhyaya*, self-study. Self-study is the act of reflection in order to deepen our understanding of thoughts and feelings. When we know what is true for us and get clear on what makes us happy and fulfilled, we align with who we are and live fully in a way that is meaningful. Svadhyaya ensures we are being the person we want to be in the world by bringing awareness to our actions and how they affect others. This upholds our integrity so we show up in a way that feels good.

Because our culture celebrates accomplishments and getting as much done as possible, pausing to reflect may seem like a waste of time, but we save energy in the end if we are confident about what to give ourselves to from the start. We become more connected to how we live when we share who we really are instead of molding ourselves into an image of who we think we should be.

I'll bet, just like me, you have found yourself in a job or relationship that wasn't right for you from the start, and when you realized it later, you thought, *How on earth did I get here*?! You got there because you weren't listening. You weren't checking in with your heart or picking up on the signals groaning from inside your gut. Or maybe you knew it wasn't right and you swallowed the truth, hoping the feeling would go away or decided you should feel differently than you did. Should is a life-killer. Should is comprised of not trusting yourself, of empowering someone else's ideas about how you ought to live. If no one has to be in your life but you, why would you let anyone else call the shots? We must be mindful of what we hold ourselves to and be conscious decision makers of our own destiny. If we aren't careful, the voice inside our head might say, "You should take that Director promotion. It will be good for your resume," even if it means longer days and time away from family or jogging or whatever it is you enjoy doing when you aren't working. If your soul is yearning for the promotion, go for it. But if it just pays more and is a boost to your ego, you might want to reconsider your motives.

A regular practice of Svadhyaya develops an awareness so keen that we listen to our instincts and stop putting ourselves in situations that make us unhappy or unfulfilled. When we trust and honor what it is we really want, we give ourselves a better chance of getting what we want. We are more likely to succeed when we do what we love and share who we are. It may lead to a better title or more money but more importantly, knowing who we are gives us distinct personality, purpose, and attracts our desires.

In moments of frustration or confusion, Svadhyaya can be an anchor. Being still and quiet can center the mind so it can think. It's not always easy to sit in the truth of our questions and answers, but bravely befriending our observations gives us information about what we need to adjust, stick out, or do. We might need to change a behavior or the dynamics of a relationship but before we do anything, we should consider all sides of a decision.

So how do we get still and listen? We stop being so busy. We hear what we say to others and notice the results of our actions. We meditate. Journal. Go for a walk. Turn off the TV and keep social commitments to a minimum. We meet up with ourselves like we would a friend and ask how we're doing. We shouldn't self-medicate or alter the mind with alcohol or other distractions when we check in like this so we are clearheaded and present.

Another great way to practice Svadhyaya is to use something we do regularly like ride a bike, drive, cook, etc. to get to know ourselves better. By bringing awareness to an activity we frequently do, we can observe our habits, shortcuts, or patterns. How we do one thing is how we do anything, and we can use this principle to notice our behaviors and amend or enhance them so we engage in activities in the way we want. For example, when I practice yoga, I tend to stick to what I know and deter new postures, just as I play it safe in life and shy away from taking risks. The yoga mat is a great place for me to explore this habit so I can be mindful and adventurous when I step off it. Having awareness of how I do things helps me be a person I feel good being. If I want to be patient, loving, and generous, I make sure that's how I'm practicing on my mat, and then I take those qualities into the smallest gestures of my day-to-day actions.

We have the power to be who we already are by removing all the crud that gets piled on top. Through stillness, becoming clear, and knowing ourselves, we make informed decisions that reflect who we are at the core.

Practice on the Mat

Svadhyaya makes the mat a mirror. Observe patterns, habits, tendencies, and transitions between postures.

<u>Suggested One-Hour Asana Practice with a Focus on Observation</u>
A video to practice part of this sequence is available: courtneyseiberling.com/yoga

(All postures are held five breath cycles unless otherwise noted.)

Intention: *Use the yoga practice to notice habits.*
Child's Pose (press third eye to the mat)
Cat/Cow (repeat five times)
Sunbird to Awkward Airplane (each side)
Down Dog
Dolphin (one minute)
Down Dog (10 breath cycles)
Tiger to Warrior One to Humble Warrior to Down Dog (each side)
Child's Pose
Warrior Two (10 breath cycles) to Triangle to Half-moon to Forward Fold (each side)
Chair Twist (each side)
Tree (without using the hand to get the leg up) to extend the leg forward to Warrior Three (each side)

Legs up the Wall (three minutes)
Camel at the Wall
Upward Facing Bow or Superman
Seated Wide-legged Forward Fold
Double Pigeon (two minutes each side)
Seated Forward Fold
Forward Fold Twist over Bolster (each side)
Child's Pose over Bolster (switch to other cheek)
Corpse (five to eight minutes)
Easy Seat: two-minute meditation

Consideration

Can you be aware of your habits? Do they reflect who you want to be?

Mantra

Pause to observe.

Personal Account

I hate conflict. I want to resolve friction as soon as it is felt so I don't have to worry about someone being mad at me, and I go out of my way to make sure no one is. I loathe the space of the unknown and am quick to come to conclusions to avoid feeling unsettled or unsure even though I know feeling unsettled and unsure is a part of life. Rushing outcome is dangerous and making decisions before understanding how we really feel doesn't help us make the right ones. It is easy to mask anxiety with quick fixes to alleviate discomfort or to play it safe to feel secure, but acting out of fear multiplies problems and limits possibilities.

I made a mess when I broke up with a long-term boyfriend and started a relationship with a man I barely knew. My boyfriend and I had recently bought a house together and in the height of huge conversations about how we wanted to cohabitate, whether we wanted to have kids, and our future, I left and started dating someone new. It devastated my boyfriend. It shocked our friends. It confused our parents, and as I was moving out and trying to put a new life together, I kept thinking, *Just go back to the old one and say you're sorry and be happy and comfortable for the rest of your life*.

But I knew I couldn't. Things weren't right with my boyfriend and even though it was going to be hard for a while, I knew it would be better later when I was in my own place and able to fully explore a relationship with this other man. He seemed more right for me. I kept telling myself this as I hauled heavy boxes around and slept on a friend's couch, while my finances crept into debt, when I took the wrong freeway home because I'd forgotten where I lived, and as I explained my reasoning to all the people who had once thought I was the kindest, most thoughtful person in the world.

As it turned out, I was more in sync with the new guy than my former boyfriend. I could be myself around him, and our priorities were similar. But then guilt set in. And then doubt. I hurt a man I'd committed myself to, and I missed him. I wondered if I made a mistake and confused comfort for immobility. Had I run away at the first sign of conflict? Wanted him to be someone he wasn't? Been through too much change too fast? I mourned the qualities my ex had that my new boyfriend didn't and craved the security that came from knowing someone so well.

During the holidays, I freaked out. I told my new boyfriend I wanted to get back together with my former one. I called my ex-boyfriend and said I was wrong and could we try again? He was surprisingly game. For a day or two, it felt so right to be back in the presence of our familiar love. I was safe. But after a few days, there I was, fighting for him to see my version of our future while he was asking for reassurance he could trust me. We were having two separate conversations like they were the same. All those fears of being misaligned resurfaced and that feeling crawled back up inside me again and was so unbearable that I made another panicked decision.

I left for the second time. It felt especially cruel this round. The guilt was worse than before because now I'd hurt two men. I needed to do better and be better, to stop acting out of reaction, and even though I so badly wanted to call the man who was more right for me and tell him I wanted to give it another go, I didn't. I spent every minute trying not to text him because I knew in order to get myself out of this mess, I had to sit in the mess and figure out what was going on with me. I needed to practice Svadhyaya.

I started to observe my thoughts. I wrote them down in my journal and told myself not to worry about what I wrote or how anyone else would feel about it. I didn't make plans or feel obligated to talk to anyone about what was happening in my life. Instead, I meditated. I did yoga. I noticed my patterns without judgment. It sounds peaceful, but it was hell. Being alone with my thoughts was uncomfortable and scary. Admitting I may not have either of these men ever again brought great sadness. I was nervous with time, they'd each meet someone else, and I'd be alone forever. Solitude felt like a nowhere-land, but then something came flying at me like a dart:

You are punishing yourself.

I was. I was punishing myself for making a decision that hurt someone else, but I was really punishing myself for not going after what I wanted. I wanted the man who I dated after I left my boyfriend and the house, but I wouldn't let myself have him. I confused missing my ex-boyfriend for guilt. I muddled loving my ex with being able to create a life with him. I prioritized what I thought I should do over what I needed to do to be happy.

I only took a shallow dive into Svadhyaya, but I felt revived. I reached out to the man I wanted to be with, and he agreed to meet me at a bar that evening. As soon as he walked through the door, I let him into my arms in the way I'd wanted to take him before. We celebrated our birthdays together, and I spent time with his family on Thanksgiving, but then feelings for my ex reemerged. Even though I wanted to be with this man, I wasn't ready for a new relationship. I couldn't open my heart again just yet.

One Friday evening while taking a tango lesson together, the man I wanted and I couldn't find our groove. We were stepping on each other's feet, turning at the wrong times, and he was trying to lead, but I wouldn't let him. We stumbled over each other for a few more songs before he threw his hands up in the air and exclaimed, "I feel like us dancing together is a metaphor for how our entire relationship has been: totally out of sync."

He was right. He had been patient and ready to have a relationship with me, but I wasn't letting him have one. We walked off the dance floor and around the block several times, speaking more honest and open with one another than we'd ever been.

The next morning, we broke up. It was horribly sad but also a relief. Maybe he could finally find what he deserved: a woman who was ready to be there, and I could stop pressuring myself to be that woman. Perhaps I could devote myself to getting over my ex and get clear on who I was after that relationship. This time, I spent months alone hiking, listening to music, writing…hours and hours, weekends where I didn't see anyone, solo dinners wining and dining myself. It was such a reprieve not to have to show up to anyone else. I could just be me. I saw who I was without a relationship after two very difficult ones, and I let myself know feelings of anxiety, sadness, and fear. As I did, the unease dissipated, and my best qualities resurfaced. I remembered what was important to me and how I wanted to spend my time. I reengaged with what mattered and started sharing this beauty with those around me. I was present for the first time in the longest time. I was cracking jokes and experiencing real joy again. It felt good. Damn good. Here I was: the person who I thought had left, healed from time to herself, appreciative for what she learned from her last two relationships, open and ready to love again, whenever love was ready for her.

Your Turn (to journal)

Transcribe the dialogue of a conversation you had today. Study your part as if you were a character in a play. Do you like the character? Would you change any lines?

10 **ISHVARA PRANIDHANA** – WONDER

The best moments in life are the simplest – the ones we can't plan for. They include sunlight sorting its way through the branches of a tree, a symphony of wind, an impromptu game of peek-a-boo with a toddler, or a welcomed conversation with a stranger at a coffee shop. These moments don't happen unless we open ourselves and allow them to happen. We can easily sink into routines or walk with our heads down in our phones and wonder why we feel unfulfilled or unseen. Life doesn't open to us unless we open to life, and life is not inherently meaningful. We must make it so, and we do this by choosing to see the world's magnificence.

Ishvara pranidhana, wonder, is the last of the Niyamas and is a celebration of the spiritual. When we look for wonder around us and revel in it, we awaken our spirit. Wonder is childlike, and this Niyama is all about seeing the world in the way a child does – with curiosity and awe. We can build our wonder skills by noticing the beauty around us: the softness of a dog's fur, a cactus blooming, or the clear blue hue of the sky. Lighting a candle before yoga can make a practice feel more intentional. Starting the day with a meditation or poem can remind us of our beating heart. Taking a moment to look into the eyes of someone we love and tell them how important they are puts us in relationship with the divine.

Looking back on the day, it's always the small things that stick, not the accomplishments, milestones, or tasks checked off a to-do list. Life can be monotonous and boring if we aren't active participants in it. We can lack purpose if we don't fill our days with a focus or become exhausted by responsibility if we don't take responsibility for our own happiness. Most of our busyness is a decoy — a distraction from having to be present or intimate. Keeping busy might make us feel as though we are engaging, but it really just prevents us from being in our breath, the moment, or an experience, and being any of these places is an opportunity to settle into real joy. There is magic in the mundane, but we must look for it.

What we call "coincidences" can also be moments of Ishvara pranidhana like when we run into someone at the grocery store we've been meaning to call or a song comes on the radio that's just the one we needed to hear. Seeing signs we're on the right path offers confirmation or encouragement, and when we align with our true intentions, they happen.

Ishvara pranidhana is sometimes translated as "surrendering to a higher source." This means we honor something larger than ourselves overseeing the course of our lives and uniting us with everything else (like God, but

God doesn't have to be a religious thing). Acknowledging this greatness allows us to give in to the mystery of life so we don't have to have all the answers and yet somehow, we feel more inclined to seek them. Instead of getting wrapped up in our individual concerns and feeling separate, offering ourselves to a higher source shows us the bigger picture and petty perspectives fall away.

We can practice awe and surrender by bringing awareness to our breath. Recognize what a miracle it is. Breath is our life force, and the body breathes itself all day without us consciously having to do anything. Notice how you are breathing. Drop in to deep, gentle, steady breaths. If there is tension in the body, draw your attention there and use the breath to soften and release it. Allow the breath to flow in and out like an ocean tide, really taking in the element of air on the inhale and grounding down to the earth on the exhale. Stay here for as many cycles as feels good. When you are done with the exercise, notice if anything has shifted since you began it. My guess is that you feel in union within yourself and everything around you. You've surrendered. Look around. Welcome to Ishvara pranidhana.

Practice on the Mat

Make a sacred space to honor the practice. Light a candle. Dim the lights. Play beautiful music. Treat the body as a temple and worship it with slow movements and steady breath. Embody Ishvara pranidhana, wonder.

Suggested One-Hour, Heart Opening and Forward Folding Asana Practice, Using Movement as a Ritual

A video to practice part of this sequence is available: courtneyseiberling.com/yoga

(All postures are held seven breath cycles unless otherwise noted.)

Intention: *Make practice sacred today. Slow down your breath and movements.*

Child's Pose: *Take interest in the miracle of the breath.* (10 breath cycles, then open knees wider and 10 more breath cycles.)

Rabbit

Cobra (repeat five times)

Superman (repeat three times, rest cheek down to the side between sets)

Down Dog with Twist (each side)

Forward Fold

Mountain Pose to Cactus (repeat three times)

Moon (repeat two times each side)

Sun A – arms up, Forward Fold, halfway lift, Forward Fold, arms up, hands in prayer at heart (repeat three times)

Sun B – Chair, Forward Fold, halfway lift, Forward Fold, Plank, Down Dog, Warrior One, Plank, Down Dog (repeat each side three times, hold each pose in the first set for 10 breath cycles)

Lizard to Half-split (each side)

Warrior One to Humble Warrior (each side)

Dancer (each side)

Legs up the Wall (three minutes)

Hero with Shoulder Opener (each side)

Bridge (repeat three times)

Reclined Twist (each side)
Double Pigeon (two minutes each side)
Head-to-Knee (each side)
Seated Forward Fold
Single Pigeon (two minutes each side)
Corpse (five to eight minutes)

Consideration

Can you make moments in your life more ceremonious and special? When you drink a glass of water, can you feel it clean and cool on your throat? Can you stop and smell flowers on your walk? Take a deep breath? Touch your lover's face?

Mantra

Open to possibility.

Personal Account

I woke up on the anniversary of my father's death unsure how to commemorate it. I considered a long hike or going to a concert but neither felt quite right, and the morning hours slipped away. I messaged my mother and my brother that I loved them. I had a call with my life coach. I drank coffee, researched a supplement I was considering, and then stopped to do the math — it had been 20 years since my father's passing. I couldn't believe it. Twenty years. I'd lived more of my life without my dad than with him.

Dumbfounded at the dining room table, I put on an album and stared out the window at an adjacent apartment building, the rattle of air conditioners conducting a concerto of noise. I felt even more pressure to make it special knowing it was such a big anniversary.

Two more albums slinked by, and my boyfriend asked if I wanted to go out for lunch. I was hungry and agreed, threw on a hat, and upgraded my tank top to a clean one but was still in some variation of my pajamas. I brushed my teeth as my boyfriend searched Yelp for lunch spots. He'd recently moved to a new neighborhood, and we were having fun exploring it.

"How about this place?" he asked and handed me his phone.

Heritage was the name of the cafe. I swiped the photos on the app. The restaurant was quaint with tall ceilings and natural light, and large stacks of leafy greens were pictured on white plates.

"Perfect," I said, and tapped the map to direct us.

The moment we arrived, I regretted my decision not to dress in actual clothes. Other customers wore their Saturday brunch best. The restaurant was small, light curving down from the Mason jar lamps above. A baby shower was showering over a large table near the entrance, and little old ladies were dressed to the nines with their hair sprayed in waves, nails the same shade as their sweater sets.

A gentleman in a beret asked how many we were, and I

held up two fingers. We followed him to a table in the middle of the restaurant, and I flapped a folded napkin from the place setting onto my sweatpant-ed lap. Another man brought us fresh bread and hummus on a wood panel. He looked like the brother of the man who'd seated us, the two tag-teaming all the tables in the restaurant with skill and grace. My boyfriend and I ordered rosewater lemonade and were brought large jars of it, blackberries and mint springs floating on top of pink liquid. We each selected a salad: one with roasted vegetables and beets, the other a spicy corn and cauliflower medley.

After a few gifts from the baby shower table were unwrapped and googled over, a woman appeared from the back with our salads. She looked like the sister of the two waiters. *How sweet*, I thought. *A family establishment.* The woman's skin glowed with kindness, not of youth or creams, and she was tailored neatly in black. I couldn't take my eyes from her pink-glazed lips as she asked if we'd been to the restaurant before. We shook our heads no and said it was our first time.

"Your first time? Welcome!" she exclaimed.

I asked her name, and she said it was Elisa. It fit her. Elisa told us to enjoy the salads and fluttered back to the kitchen to prepare the next order. One of the brothers came around to refill our jars even though the menu said there were no free refills. We finished what we could of the oversized salads and asked for the check, though what showed up next was not the bill, but Elisa.

She placed a small, scalloped dish in front of us and sweetly sang, "Complimentary dessert for the happy couple," and then scurried back to the kitchen.

The dessert was a custard of some kind. Chocolate. I lifted a small spoon and took a bite: rice pudding, light and chewy. Tears welled up in my eyes, and my hand dropped down to the table.

"What's wrong?" my boyfriend asked.

"Rice pudding was my father's favorite. A stranger brought me my father's favorite dessert on the 20th anniversary of his death."

My boyfriend raised his eyebrows in a sentimental acknowledgement. I told him the story my family tells about my dad as a kid, and how one evening, he wouldn't finish his dinner. My grandmother, overcome with frustration, dumped an entire bowl of rice pudding over his head. There's a photo of it: my dad is screaming, the gooey, gloppy chocolate dripping down his ears. In time, my father would come to love rice pudding, but the picture says otherwise.

Elisa came to check on us during my gushy consumption of the rice pudding, and I tugged at her sweater sleeve. "I don't mean to make this sad, but I have to tell you something. Today is the 20th anniversary of my father's death and there's this thing with him and rice pudding and look what you've brought me," I warbled, motioning to the half-eaten dessert.

Elisa put her hands over her heart. "In Armenia," she said, "it is a tradition to make the deceased's favorite food on the day of their death to honor them. On the anniversary of my father's death, we serve complimentary feta wrapped in lavash with olive oil in the restaurant."

Tears spun in my eyes again. I knew what a special moment I was sharing with this special stranger and how she was offering a way to acknowledge a day I didn't know how to honor. My boyfriend and I finished the rice pudding, paid the bill, and just as we were about to leave, Elisa appeared again with a purse over her arm.

"I wanted to say goodbye," she said. "My mother is sick, and I have to fly east to see her. I'm on my way to the airport."

A tender arrow struck my heart. I knew what it was like to have a sick parent. I told Elisa how sorry I was to hear her mother was ill and how much I appreciated her being a part of this day. We hugged, soft check against soft cheek, this beautiful gift from the Universe in my arms, our fathers somewhere both near and far.

Your Turn (to journal)

What was magnificent today?

APPLICATION

Change doesn't happen overnight. Steady intention causes change. The shifts you've experienced of me in these essays were gradual, and any wisdom came from years of making conscious efforts to consider things in different ways.

The Yamas and Niyamas are a place I can land when I feel myself starting to crash or a way to unstick myself when I'm stuck, and I hope you experience this of them, too. If not, I'd encourage you to find a system to consult whenever you feel lost, anxious, or discouraged.

Shifts happen when we bring awareness to our thoughts and take responsibility for our own actions. I have to make room in my body first, which clears up space in my mind so I can see situations with a fresh perspective. Yoga is my practice for wholeness, but yoga isn't the only one. Anything that gets the mind aware of the breathing and the breath supporting the physical body can settle and embolden us.

Here are some suggestions of how to use this book, but please take liberties to reference it however you like:

Teachers

Offer a ten-class series on the Yamas and Niyamas, using each instruction to focus on one of the principles. Teach the Mantra and Asana Practice from the chapter or make up your own. End with the Consideration.

If you have a weekly class of semi-regular students, spend a month on each principle and work the same sequence for several sessions so students really start to understand the concept in their bodies.

Students

Consider each principle for a month (a month of truth, a month of gratitude, a month of keeping spaces clean, etc.) Write the Mantra for the principle on a Post-it and stick it to your bathroom mirror to remind you. Apply the concept to as many parts of your day as possible. Really respond to the journal prompts. Really do the yoga sequences. Really reflect and notice your thoughts.

Write each principle on an index card and have the stack of cards at the ready. Whenever you feel frustrated, trapped, or sad, grab the stack of cards and decide which principle you could apply to the situation or feeling you are experiencing. Go back and reread that section of the book. Apply it.

***

A reminder: life is a practice. These concepts are a reset button. Every moment is a new opportunity to decide who you want to be and how you want to show up. If you mess up, try again.

Resource

Yoga workout videos to physically practice the Yamas and Niyamas are available:
courtneyseiberling.com/yoga

Hire Courtney

Courtney is available to facilitate workshops on the Yamas and Niyamas at yoga studios or to lead philosophy modules for yoga teacher training programs. For inquiries:
courtneyseiberling.com

(WITH) GRATITUDE

Daniel, Stacey, my family, Marielle, Tarabu, Cally, Faithy, Cory, Aric, Trent, Niko, Marty, Alex, Carol, Samantha, Ellen, Lisa, Judy, Songhi, Tony, Leo, Shahbano, Joe, Gary, Jamie, Monica, Cyndy, Kristen, Cindy, Julie, Regina, Kali, Bonnie, Kathleen, Margaret, Brandon, Tim, Nick, my East Village Yoga gals, and Drew

You are all my greatest teachers and cheerleaders. Thank you for showing up in a big way.